COMING HOME

COMING HOME

From Grief to Growth:
A true story

EBONIE STIRLING-GATT

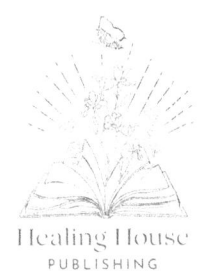

Healing House
PUBLISHING

First Published in Australia in 2024
by Healing House Publishing
www.healinghousepublishing.com

The National Library of Australia Cataloguing-in-Publication entry:

Title: Coming Home
Sub title: From Grief to Growth: A True Story
Author: Ebonie Stirling-Gatt
Paperback ISBN: 978-0-6485478-5-3

Editor: Vanessa Barrington
Cover and Internal Design: Heidi Glasson

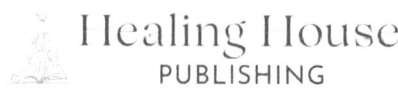

Healing House
PUBLISHING

AUTHOR DISCLAIMER

This memoir contains sensitive content, including topics of suicide, disordered eating and childhood trauma.

It is a work of creative non-fiction.

The events, timelines, and characters portrayed in this book are based on real experiences, but some details have been adapted, changed or recreated to enhance the narrative flow. While the core of the story remains true, certain aspects have been fictionalised, adjusted or reimagined for storytelling purposes.

If you or someone you know is struggling, please seek professional help.

Phone: Lifeline, 13 11 44 (Australia only).

To my mum,
who continues to be my guiding light,
and to my friends
who became my family.

PROLOGUE

I wrapped my arms around Maddie's shoulders and held her tight, not wanting to let her go just yet; it all felt so surreal.

"I'm going to miss you so much. I'll call you when I land. I love you," I said, releasing her from my suffocating embrace. I wiped away happy tears and began walking down the boarding corridor without looking back.

As I stood amongst the long line of people waiting to board the plane, I looked out the window beside me, took a deep breath in and smiled softly. I was about to do the one thing I never thought I'd ever be able to do. I was moving to the other side of the world with a single suitcase, a backpack and no return flight booked.

I was terrified. For the first time in my life, I had no plan, no idea where I'd be in six months or when exactly I'd see my friends again. But the freedom I felt, the excitement that was erupting inside of me as I entered this new chapter of my life, was one of the most empowering feelings in the world.

"Those who look for seashells will find seashells; those who open them will find pearls."

– Al Ghazali

1

It was a glorious summer's day, not a cloud in the sky, and the sun's rays were shining directly onto our skin. My mum was walking along the water's edge, sinking her feet into the cold, wet sand with every step, leaving behind perfectly moulded footprints almost twice the size of mine. I followed closely behind her, trying not to leave any footprints of my own by placing my tiny feet into hers instead.

Mum was carrying my orange sand bucket while she watched me skip ahead, running in and out of the water as the little waves chased me up towards the dry sand before folding back onto themselves and returning to the deep sea. I continued to run back and forth, digging around in the sand, trying to find the prettiest-looking shells for my collection. Mum and I were always on the hunt for an empty but intact pipi shell washed up on the shoreline. They had always fascinated me; a combination of Mum and my favourite colours together with their smooth pearly outer layer, lined with pink-purple bands, opening to a rich purple colour on the inside. They had more character than the other shells to me, but of course, they were always so difficult to find.

My eyes lit up as I spotted a perfectly undamaged pipi shell sitting there, waiting just for me. I picked it up and gently dusted the wet sand granules off its smooth, shiny exterior and eagerly ran towards my mum, holding it out in front of me.

"I found one, I found one!" I exclaimed.

"Woohoo! Well done, Bub!" she hooted.

I carefully placed it into the bucket, sitting it on top of the rest of the shells I had collected and asked Mum to look after it for me.

"Don't worry, it will be safe in here," she reassured me.

The beach had always been my mum's happy place, which meant it became mine, too. As soon as she arrived, she'd become the person I wanted her to be all the time. Her smile would come alive, and her crystal blue eyes would sparkle in the sunlight as she looked out to the horizon ahead of us.

Once I was satisfied with my accumulation of shells, it was time for a swim – my favourite part of the morning. Mum held my hand as we made our way through the beach breaks, walking deeper and deeper into the ocean. She pulled my arm up above my head to help lift me in the air as I jumped over the waves that were crashing into us. Eventually, we got so deep that my little legs could no longer touch the bottom, but I knew I could effortlessly float over the smooth, gentle waves with my head poking through the top.

As the cycle continued and the waves began to get slightly rougher, I slid myself in front of her. She wrapped her arms around my tiny waist, holding me tightly against her warm body.

"Ready? Three, two, one…" she said as I gripped tightly onto her and took a deep breath in before we dove through the wave together. In that moment, I felt so connected to her, both physically and emotionally. It was a feeling that I wanted to last forever.

* * * * *

Mum was often described as being quite a stunner throughout her younger adult years, with 'boys chasing after her like they were bees around a honey pot.' She was tall, slim, and had a very athletic figure from her days of playing competitive netball. Her fine, sandy blonde hair sat in waves just below her shoulders and was neatly complemented by a classic fringe that lightly covered her forehead and highlighted her sea-blue eyes and high cheekbones.

My mum always knew how to have a fun time; she loved going out with her friends and jamming out to her favourite karaoke songs, singing, and dancing the night away with a glass of champagne in her hand. She'd laugh so loud you could hear her from across the other side of the room, but it was laughter that made you want to laugh, too. Her vibrant, energetic and carefree attitude was so magnetic everyone wanted to be her friend; people were drawn to her presence.

Her eye-catching confidence meant she was usually one of the first amongst her group of friends to be asked out on a date. Sometimes, she would accept. Other times, she would deny them. It seemed the men she met didn't meet her high standards, so one day before I was born, she decided to post an ad about herself in the dating section of the Daily Bulletin.

Jan Stirling: 34 y.o, 5' 9"
I am a very down-to-earth, honest and outgoing high school
teacher who enjoys listening to live music, spending time outdoors and
going on weekend adventures. I am looking for someone similar to
share my life with.

They say there are plenty of fish in the sea but apparently, only one guy responded to her ad, which meant she didn't have a lot of choice. When she finally made the decision to contact him, he was eager to take her out on a date. They finalised the details of their first meeting over a phone call, and of course, my mum took this opportunity to find out a little more about him.

He had moved over to Australia from New Zealand during his late teenage years and was working in construction as a builder, which he'd been doing since he'd left high school. A handyman with a stable job, on a relatively decent wage… tick, she thought. When she arrived at their meeting spot and saw him walking towards her, she immediately noticed his lean, muscular figure was slightly taller than hers. His golden-brown, olive-toned complexion was quite the contrast to her rather fair, freckly skin. As he got closer, she saw he had a well-defined jawline and short but dense black hair, paired with noticeably thick, bushy eyebrows. When she looked into his smiling, chocolate-coloured eyes, she couldn't help but feel the butterflies dancing around in her stomach. Physical attraction… tick, tick!

She soon learnt that his father was of European descent, having migrated to New Zealand from Malta in his early twenties, hence the darker features. Most of his immediate family – his mother, father and younger sister – were still living in New Zealand, while his older brother had moved over to Western Australia. He stayed in close contact with his family, especially his mum, but unfortunately, they didn't see each other all that often.

Their first date went better than she had expected. He made her laugh until her cheeks hurt; he was witty but sensible and made her feel safe and comfortable in his company, all of which were important factors to her… tick, tick and, tick! After spending more quality time getting to know each other and realising that he had successfully ticked most of her boxes, she began to fall for him fairly quickly. The loved-up couple got married in 1998, and in January of 1999, I entered the world as a chunky eight-pound, thirteen-ounce baby girl with almost a full head of black hair. From that moment on, I became their pride and joy.

* * * * *

As a child, the connection I shared with my dad was like no other bond I'd ever had. He absolutely adored me – I was his princess, and he was my hero.

I sat on his lap and put my tiny, cold hands onto his warm cheeks, looked directly into his dark, glossy brown eyes and whispered, "I wish I could marry you, Dad."

The top of his cheeks lifted as he let out a gentle chuckle, "You'll find your prince charming one day, Bub." I swear my parents called me Bub more than my given name.

He was always so playful and loved to joke around with me at any opportunity he got. On most days when he arrived home from work, he knew I'd be hiding, waiting for him to find me.

"I wonder where Ebonie could be," he'd say aloud as he strolled into my room and began his search for me. I'd predictably crouch down in the corner of my wardrobe tucked in behind my hanging clothes, with the door slightly ajar, giggling to myself as I watched him look for me under my bed, behind the curtains, and in my clothes drawers. This would continue until I thought it was time to reveal myself from my dark, squishy hiding spot. I'd jump out and shout, "I'm here!"

"Oh, you're too good at this game!" he'd reply, catching me as I jumped into his arms.

I looked up to him in many ways. He was a good dad, and he taught me a lot. Mostly the more outdoorsy, hands-on kind of stuff like learning how to ride a bike without training wheels, how to roller skate and remain upright, or how to use a power drill without splitting the wood under the screw.

Once I had the bicycle down pat, he thought he'd take it up a notch and teach me how to ride a unicycle. So, at the age of five, I successfully learnt how to ride one, and my future aspiration was to join the circus.

I liked that he always encouraged me to have a go, no matter how difficult the task seemed. Even if I failed, he would encourage me to get back up and try again. That was the kind of relationship we had.

"The walls we build around us to keep sadness out also keep out the joy."

– Jim Rohn

2

My parent's relationship had its ups and downs, as do most but it seemed to reach a point where the tough times began to outweigh the good. I watched Mum as she stood at the kitchen bench, chopping up vegetables for dinner. My Dad walked up behind her and wrapped his arms around her waist. She stopped what she was doing and pushed his hands away.

"Please don't, I'm busy," she snapped. Saddened by her immediate rejection, my dad quickly took a step back and stood there for a moment before walking out of the kitchen without a single word. I could see he was trying to maintain some form of connection with my mum, but for some reason, she was not willing to accept it.

As I grew older, the hostility between my parents intensified. The arguing became a constant occurrence I couldn't escape. The tension became unbearable; the house was often deadly quiet, and I'd ache to turn on the television just to lighten the mood a little. One day, after a particularly bad fight, I decided it was up to me to make it better.

I walked to the other end of the house into my dad's room and found him sitting on the edge of his bed with his head resting heavily in his hands. For as long as I had remembered, my parents never slept in the same bed. Whenever I'd asked why, the best answer I got was that they loved each other but it was just a different kind of love… whatever that meant!

I hadn't ever seen my dad look so sad and frustrated all at once. I gently sat on the bed beside him with my legs hanging off the edge.

"What happened between you and Mum?"

He reluctantly lifted his head to look at me. "Don't worry, Bub, it's nothing."

Being the persistent five-year-old I was, I continued to question him. "But why are you so angry at each other? I don't like it when you fight," I said softly, looking down at my feet dangling in the air.

"Eb, I'm sorry for arguing with your mum in front of you, but we just need some time apart."

I propped myself up onto his bed and wrapped my little arms around his shoulders.

"Okay. Well, I love you," I said, using his body as a springboard to help me jump off the edge of the bed and walk out of his room.

I went straight to Mum, hoping she could give me some more answers. She was sitting at the dining room table, staring down at her feet. Her slumped posture was not the reassurance I was searching for. She could tell I was distressed, but nothing she said was making me feel any better.

"Thank you for trying to help Bub, but it's time for bed now. Tomorrow is a new day. There is no need to worry about your dad and me," she immediately started, trying to reassure me.

I realised that evening there was nothing I could do to fix the situation. This wasn't the only time I found myself wandering up and down the house, getting as much as I could out of one parent to then go and tell the other, hoping it would help in some way. It never did.

* * * * *

The house always felt so empty. It was dull and miserable. I really didn't like being there.

"What's wrong with mum?" I asked my dad one day after returning home from school. I was confused. Why had she suddenly shut herself in her room at four o'clock in the afternoon?

"She's just not feeling well today, Eb," he shrugged.

I walked towards her bedroom door and slowly opened it without knocking. She was tucked under the covers, lying so still, curled up in the foetal position, and although the curtains were closed, the sun continued to shine its light into the darkness. I made my way to the side of her bed and sat on the edge so I could see her face. She reluctantly opened her eyes and took a deep breath in like she'd just woken up from a deep sleep.

"Mum? Are you okay?" I whispered.

"I've just got a headache this afternoon, Eb and I'm not feeling myself," she mumbled, closing her eyes again. I gently touched her shoulder.

"Are you going to get up soon?" I pleaded. I wanted my fun, bubbly mum to return.

"I'll see how I feel; otherwise, Dad will cook your dinner," she said. It felt like she had shut me down instantly without any further consideration.

I kissed her on the cheek, slid myself off the bed and closed the door quietly behind me.

* * * * *

On the evening that everything fell apart, emotions were flying left, right and centre, along with many harsh words and plenty of slammed doors. I sat on the couch in the lounge room, hugging my knees close to my chest, listening to the chaos unravelling around me.

"I don't want you here anymore. I want you to leave tonight!" My mum shouted

"It'll be my pleasure; I couldn't stand another night in this house with you!" Dad barked back.

The pure anger my parents had towards each other was like nothing I had ever witnessed before. I got up off the couch and walked timidly towards Dad's room. I stood quietly outside his door and watched as he packed up as much stuff as he could fit into his large black duffle bag. I knew he was leaving. I didn't know where he was going or whether he was coming back, but all I wanted to know was when I was going to see him again.

I followed closely behind him as he rushed out the front door towards his ute. He turned around to see me looking straight up at him with sad, glassy eyes. He took a deep breath.

"Eb, I promise I will see you very soon. Everything will be okay.

I love you." He was choking up, trying to hold back his tears. They had both kept telling me not to worry that everything would be okay, but nothing about this felt okay. He hopped in the ute and pushed his keys in the ignition to insinuate it was time for him to go. I took a step back, allowing him to shut his car door. He didn't look at me again. He couldn't. I stood at the bottom of the driveway, tears streaming down my face as I watched his car drive off, leaving me behind.

"I'd love to take a tour inside the darkness that fills your mind. I'd try to find the light. I'd show you all the magical things you've forgotten and left behind."

– Moomer

3

After my parents split up, Dad moved into an old, run-down two-bedroom house that he had previously started renovating in Brisbane, about an hour north of Mum's place. The legal arrangement was that I would live with Mum during the week and visit Dad on the weekends, and although I didn't get much of a say in the matter, it was the most convenient option for everyone involved in terms of school and extracurricular activities.

I always looked forward to the quality time I got to spend with Dad. Our weekends together were for no one else but me and him, jam-packed with all the activities that I rarely got to do when I was with Mum. He'd take me out to the pub for dinner just so that I could play in the kids' room, even if that meant he'd be left at the dining table on his own, or we'd get my favourite Indian takeout and watch 'Around the Twist' on television until I fell asleep in his bed.

On Sunday mornings, we'd get up early to go to the markets and get Poffertjes (mini-Dutch pancakes) for breakfast before going to the park, where I'd climb any tree I could manage to get myself up. I'd have so much fun with him that I'd struggle to return home to the same quiet, miserable, and gloomy environment Mum's house was.

He poured all of his attention into me and made me feel like I was the most important person in his world because I was, and I was regularly reminded of this. He wrote me a card once, for no rhyme or reason. It was probably one of the most special messages he had ever written to me.

Dear Ebonie,
I was on my lunch break today, walking through the shops, and I saw
this card with beautiful reds and purples (our colours together).
I want you to know that I miss you, and I love you so much.
You're the most special person in my life.
Don't ever forget that.
You can ring me any time you want to, ok?
All my love forever
Daddy xx

* * * * *

About two years after the divorce, my dad sat me down to explain that he had a new female friend in his life who he had been spending a lot of his spare time with. Her name was Julie, she had two children, but really, the only thing I cared about was that the drive to her place was two and a half hours away from my mum, something I instantly felt anxious about. He wanted me to meet her, so I reluctantly agreed to go with him one weekend.

When we first arrived, I was introduced to Julie's daughter, who was about one year younger than me, and her son, who was a couple of years older. Being in a completely new and unfamiliar environment with a family whom I had only just met made me feel anxious. I wasn't overly thrilled to be staying the night. It didn't take long to develop a deep-rooted feeling of jealousy about my dad spending quality time with another woman, and it made me behave in ways that, as a child, I struggled to control.

* * * * *

I lay on one of the blow-up mattresses that Julie had set up for us in the living room downstairs. The movie we were watching had just finished, and the other two had fallen asleep. Meanwhile, I was wide awake, staring at the ceiling, beginning to feel more and more uneasy. I just needed to see my dad. I slowly removed the blanket from my legs and shuffled my way towards the edge of the bed, careful not to disturb the others. I quietly walked through the kitchen and up the spiral staircase, heading towards Julie's bedroom.

Is that them I can hear, or is it just the television playing? Please, please, just let it be a movie.

I stood silently outside their door, listening to the moaning. I was almost certain it was too real to be a movie. My stomach dropped to the floor, and I felt like I was going to be sick. I couldn't find the courage to interrupt them, but I also couldn't stand to listen any longer. I slowly stepped away from the door to go back down the stairs before noticing my dad's bag sitting on the kitchen counter. Using the moonlight that was shining rather brightly through the glass windows, I began to rummage my way through my dad's things, praying he'd left his phone in his bag.

Ah, thank goodness, it's here.

I dialled Mum's number, one of the only numbers I'd successfully memorised by heart, hoping she would answer even though it was very late.

"Hello?" she murmured, just as it was about to go to message bank. I had clearly just woken her up.

"Mum, it's me," I whispered. The muscles in my throat began to tighten as I tried to stop myself from crying and continue. "I can't sleep. Dad and Julie are in their bedroom upstairs, and I'm too scared to knock on their door. I don't want to be here." My breath was becoming short and sharp, and I could feel my heart thumping against my chest.

"Eb, it's late, you can't come home now. You will be okay. Just go and tell your dad you can't sleep. He will stay with you," she assured.

"Okay," I mumbled, disappointed by her response.

"You'll be fine, Eb. I will see you tomorrow. I love you."

"I love you too." I put the phone back in his bag and briefly contemplated what to do next. A few minutes later, I found myself back upstairs, waiting nervously and instantly regretting my decision to knock on their door. Just as I was about to turn around to walk in the opposite direction, I heard the door unlock.

The door slowly opened, and my eyes darted to see Julie scrambling to cover herself up in bed behind Dad.

Shit. The noise I'd heard earlier was definitely not coming from the television.

"Eb, are you okay? What's wrong?" he asked in a complete frazzle, trying his best to deter my attention away from Julie.

"I'm sorry, I can't sleep," I apologised looking down at my feet.

He sighed and opened the door a little wider and stepped aside as if to invite me in.

"Come lay with us for a while."

I tucked myself under the covers and turned to lay on my side as my dad cradled me in his arms from behind while Julie lay on the other side of him.

I felt slightly less panicked than I had been feeling five minutes ago, but also uncomfortable with how awkward I had made the current situation.

I allowed my dreary eyes to close, trying to drift off to sleep, but all I could focus on were the whispers happening behind me. Selfishly, in that moment, I just wanted all of my dad's attention on me. I could tell neither of them wanted me there.

I opened my eyes to see the bright red light from the digital clock sitting on the bedside table, staring at me. 3:35am. More than an hour had gone by, and I was still no closer to falling asleep. I felt like a complete nuisance and knew I had absolutely outstayed my welcome.

This night felt like it had gone on forever, and I was now in Julie's daughter's bedroom, which was conveniently connected to Julie's room via the bathroom.

"If you need to use the toilet, I will leave the door unlocked, so you don't need to worry about knocking," Julie told me in a way that felt like she didn't want me to bother them again.

"Goodnight," Dad gently kissed my forehead before following Julie out of the room, shutting the door behind them.

I laid on my back as stiff as a plank of wood with my eyes tightly closed, breathing deeply in and out, praying the sun would make an appearance sometime soon, just so I could be a little closer to going home.

My attempt to independently fall asleep was rudely interrupted by a sudden urge to pee. I quickly got up and tip-toed towards the bathroom door before realising that it was locked.

She lied to me, I thought.

Although it was probably an accident, I couldn't help but think she had done this on purpose, to be deceitful and make me feel even more of an inconvenience than I already did. I was not going to be the one to bother them again, so I decided to use the other bathroom instead.

I eventually fell asleep and when I woke up later that morning, I dreaded having to walk downstairs and see them both. I nervously walked into the kitchen to see them preparing a cooked breakfast for everyone. My dad looked at me with sheer disappointment in his eyes. I could tell neither of them were impressed about me ruining their night. I felt like a complete burden. I sat at the table and didn't say a word. I no longer felt welcome in that house.

I just want to get the hell out of here as soon as possible, I thought.

* * * * *

My feelings about spending the weekends with my dad had abruptly done a complete one-eighty, not because I didn't want to see him, but because it was never just him and I anymore. Our weekend plans now revolved around his new girlfriend, and it was like I was just tagging along for the ride. I never felt included or wanted, and I slowly began to feel less and less important to Dad. It felt like Julie was driving a wedge between our relationship, and it terrified me.

It was my dad's weekend again, and I was sitting outside on his back porch, in my own little world, playing with scraps of wood that he had left around the house when a dark shadow suddenly blocked the warmth of the sun shining down on my bare skin. I looked up to see my dad standing over me.

"If you come with me to Julie's house tonight, I'll give you this," he said as he waved a twenty-dollar note in my face. Although I was tempted, it wasn't enough to win me over.

"No, it's okay. I want to stay here with you," I replied, determined not to return to that house again. He let out a heavy breath of frustration, knowing his genius plan to bribe an eight-year-old with money hadn't worked. He shoved the note back in his pocket and walked away without saying another word.

Later that evening, my dad was sitting on the back deck talking to Julie on the phone, explaining to her that we wouldn't be visiting this weekend, and of course, it was my fault. When I heard him finally step inside and close the sliding door behind him, I quickly emerged from his bedroom and walked down the hallway towards the kitchen to ask if he wanted to watch a movie. I poked my head around the corner and noticed him leaning up against the bench, looking down at his feet with a glass of red wine sitting firmly in his hand. I suddenly wanted to turn around.

"Is everything okay?" I asked timidly, hoping that he was a little less angry than he had appeared. He looked up to see me standing at the doorway, his eyes quickly narrowing, full of rage.

If there was ever going to be the moment when I could physically see steam coming out of someone's ears from the anger that was building up inside of them, this was that moment. Silence filled the room as I waited for him to speak. Apparently, words weren't powerful enough to express himself. He lifted his glass towards his head and launched it across the room. Red wine splattered everywhere as the glass hit the wall and shattered to pieces.

"Go to your room!" he screamed at me. I did what I was told.

Not long after his sudden outburst, I heard the creaking of loose wooden floorboards as he walked down the hall towards my bedroom. I lay there quietly, tucked under the covers, petrified of what he was going to do or say next. He came in and sat beside me and put his hand gently on my shoulder.

"I'm sorry for yelling at you, Bub. I'm just not in a good mood tonight."

He never told me why he got so angry, and I was too scared to ask, but I knew it had something to do with what was said on the phone with Julie that evening.

He knew I didn't feel comfortable staying at her place, and he couldn't force me to go. But he also knew that she wasn't happy about the human roadblock that was interfering with their relationship, and he didn't know what to do about it.

* * * * *

Every time Dad's weekend rolled around, I'd cry to Mum, begging her not to make me go, and this became a recurring battle that never seemed to get any easier for either of us.

"Please, Mum! I don't want to go to Dad's this weekend. All he ever wants to do is go to Julie's house, and I hate it there!" I'd plead.

"Ebonie, you need to go. It is important that you keep spending time with your father," she'd reply.

One Saturday as I heard my dad's car pull up in our driveway after one of these arguments, I felt my chest suddenly tighten as the panic spread through my little body. I quickly wiped away my tears and tried to pretend to be somewhat excited to see his face. He opened the front door to see me standing there waiting for him but I watched as his smiling eyes quickly turned into a darkness that I had not seen before. My attempt to hide my distress had failed. He clenched his fists and looked in the direction of Mum, who was standing right behind me.

"It's your fault she doesn't want to come with me," he yelled at her. "You put all this shit into her head and make her think that I'm a terrible person who is incapable of being a father," he continued, his voice raising in anger.

"Jason, that's not true. I have done nothing but encourage Ebonie to see you this entire time," she said. She spoke the truth. Not once had she ever said otherwise.

He took a step towards Mum to further intimidate her with his presence.

"That's bullshit, and you know it! You're a manipulative liar, and you are brainwashing our daughter," he screamed. I could see the blood rushing to his head as his cheeks became flushed and his jaw was clenched tight.

"Jason, please stop. We don't need to do this in front of Ebonie. She is going with you, and I've already told her that," Mum pleaded.

He took a step closer to her, and she took a step back. Her body was firmly up against the wall.

"What's the point of taking her if she doesn't want to come with me?"

He lifted his arm and pointed his finger in her face.

"You're a fucking mole, and I blame you for this."

He looked deep into her eyes and took a deep breath before turning around to stop himself from doing something he was going to regret. Mum tried to hide how scared she was, but I could see straight through it. She didn't seem willing to put up a fight and stand up for herself. Maybe because she didn't want to make things worse for me, she didn't want me to witness any more than I already had. Deep down, Dad knew that it was really me who didn't want to go with him, but he didn't want to accept this. He needed someone else to blame, and Mum was the easy target.

I could see the tears building up in his eyes as he tried to control his anger, and without another word, he stormed out the front door and slammed it shut in our faces, leaving us standing there in complete shock, trying to fathom how this had all escalated so quickly.

I slowly walked towards the screen door and watched as he got back into his ute. Part of me was so relieved that he was going and leaving me behind, but another part of me wanted to chase after him and beg for forgiveness. My heart was completely torn. I heard the car engine start, and before I even had time to blink, he had pressed down so hard on the accelerator that the tyres screeched as he sped up the driveway as fast as he could.

*"Your darkest moments are only temporary, so you
must never give up on yourself when it's raining.
Your brightest moments are also temporary, so you have
to learn to live in the moment when the sun is shining."*

– Steven Bartlett

4

As a child, I noticed Mum was not like the other mums, particularly when it came to her health – she was fanatical. Everything we ate was organic, spray-free, and pesticide-free; every cleaning product or cosmetic brand we used was non-toxic and free from harsh chemicals; the water we drank was filtered, alkaline and fluoride-free. Our shoes were to be taken off at the front door; otherwise, we'd be walking pesticides and germs through the house. Seeing a conventional doctor was out of the question; Mum was convinced expensive homeopathics from her naturopath would heal any illness she had.

I remember being the one kid who sat awkwardly in the corner waiting for everyone else to get their free vaccinations at school because my mum refused to let me get mine. She had become so paranoid that she struggled to leave the house. It was like she wanted to live her life inside an imaginary bubble, protected from the outside world. If anything jeopardised that, her anxiety skyrocketed. Her extreme obsession with reaching the pinnacle of health was the very thing that drove her to become so unwell, both physically and mentally.

I had recently gotten a new nail polish set for my eighth birthday and was curious to see what the metallic rose colour looked like. I sat at my desk in my room, opened the nail polish bottle and proceeded to gently sweep the brush along the nail of my right index finger. I held my hand out in front of me and took a moment to decide if I liked the colour enough to continue, knowing that if I did, I would need to go outside. It's nice, but I can't be bothered painting the rest, I thought. I put the brush back into its bottle and tightened it closed.

It didn't take me long to realise how strong the smell of the polish really was.

Oh no, Mum is not going to be happy about this.

I decided to sit in my room for a little while longer with my door firmly shut and the window wide open, hoping it would air out before she noticed. A few moments later, there was a knock on my door.

"Ebonie, what is that smell? Have you been painting your nails in your room?" she sternly questioned as she opened the door and began to sniff the fumes through her extremely sensitive nostrils.

"No," I lied, knowing full well I had been caught.

"Don't lie to me! I can smell it," she yelled abruptly. I could see the steam coming out of her ears, and I immediately regretted my decision.

"I'm sorry, Mum, I just wanted to see the colour, that's all. I only painted one nail, see?" I pointed my finger at her to prove I was telling the truth.

"Ebonie, you know the rules. If you want to paint your nails, you need to do it outside! Now the smell has gone all through the house, and you know I can't cope with those toxic fumes!" She stormed out of my room and slammed the door in my face. I had made her so angry I was too scared to leave my room and face her.

I gave her some time to calm down, and once the smell of nail polish had finally disappeared, I slowly emerged from my room to apologise again. I quickly realised she wasn't in the house. Her bedroom was empty. She wasn't in the kitchen or watching television - I couldn't see her anywhere. I walked towards the garage and opened the door; her car was gone.

She never told me she was going out.

She never leaves the house without telling me, I thought.

My heart pounded as I started to panic. I didn't know what to do.

Why did I do that? This is all my fault, I thought.

I quickly grabbed our home phone and dialled Aunty Jan's number; the only person I knew understood Mum's random outbursts.

"Don't worry, Ebonie, I'm sure your mum wouldn't have gone far. I'll come over now to help you find her," she said when I explained what had happened.

By the time she arrived, about fifteen minutes later, Mum had returned from her sudden disappearance, pretending like nothing had happened. She was confused as to why Aunty Jan randomly turned up at our house.

"Thank you, but everything is fine Jan," she said, refusing to admit that anything was wrong.

Aunty Jan could tell how distressed I was and tried to stay for as long as she felt welcome, making general chit-chat with us before deciding it was time to leave us to figure it out for ourselves.

"Mum, I'm really sorry. I promise I won't do that again," I said, hoping she had finally forgiven me for my innocent mistake. She knelt towards me and gave me a warm hug.

"It's okay, Eb, I'm sorry for overreacting."

I could see how guilty she felt for being so irrational and blowing something so small out of proportion, but I didn't care about that anymore. I was just relieved she was home safe and not angry with me anymore.

* * * * *

She sat with her legs crossed on the cold, hard tiles with her back towards the window, her hands wrapped tightly around her hot cup of herbal tea. She gently tilted her head up towards the ceiling, closed her eyes and took a deep breath in as she felt the heat of the sun's rays shine down on the top of her forehead. I walked over to join her and watched as she slowly opened her weary eyes and forced her lips to smile as I sat down next to her.

"Eb, your life would be so much better without me in it. Can't you see that?" I could hear the desperation in her voice as she tried to convince me that this unfathomable thought was somehow true.

"No, Mum, that's not true. Can you please stop saying that?" I hated her for thinking this way, and no matter how much I tried to shut it down, the same debate continued to resurface.

"I can't keep going on like this, Eb. I'm in this deep, dark hole that I don't know how to get myself out of, and it's ruining your life," she said. I could tell she was starting to spiral.

"No, it's not!" I argued. "Why don't you try taking those tablets that are meant to help people with the same thing as you? Maybe it will be that one pill that will make it all go away," I begged her, desperate for her to try anything that could make a difference.

"No, Eb, I refuse to take any of that crap! You know that," she retorted.

"But I can't live without you, Mum; please just keep trying to get better," I said. I was trying my hardest to convince her that giving up was not the answer, that I needed her more than anyone else, and the tears began to roll down my cheeks.

I watched as her eyes suddenly lit up like she'd either seen a ghost or had some sort of brilliant idea. A flicker of hope spread through my body as I watched her put the mug of herbal tea down beside her and quickly get up from the floor. I decided to follow behind her as she swiftly walked down the hallway towards the garage.

"I'm doing it now; I can't take it anymore."

My hope was short lived. A wave of cold panic crashed over me.

"Mum, stop! What are you doing? You're scaring me!"

I stood at the doorway, watching her frantically scrummage through boxes of stuff sitting in the garage, trying to find whatever she could to supposedly end her torment. Suddenly, she stopped. She straightened up her posture and looked down at her feet, breathing heavily in exhaustion.

"Eb, please just give me some space for a few minutes."

"No, I'm not leaving you alone after what you just said!" I fought back.

"I'll be inside soon, I promise."

I was worried about what she would do if I left her alone but even more scared about what she'd do if I didn't, so I decided to trust her and slowly walked away, closing the door behind me.

"We shouldn't seek to find the ultimate right answer for ourselves, but rather, we should seek to chip away at the ways that we were wrong today that we can be a little less wrong tomorrow."

– Mark Manson

5

Mum would often lose her temper over the tiniest of things; suddenly, she'd flip a switch, and all hell would break loose as she'd chase me around the house with one hand up in the air, ready to slap me or scream at me so loud our neighbours would hear it from inside their home. Sometimes, I had no idea what I had done wrong. It was almost like simply being in the same room was enough to set her off, and for some reason, many of these outbursts would occur whilst we were driving somewhere in the car, which meant that I had no escape. I was stuck, with my seat belt fastened and nowhere to go.

One day before school around the age of eight, I sat in the passenger seat and waited nervously for her to lock the front door of the house before getting into the car. She got into the driver's seat and gripped onto the steering wheel so tightly that her fingertips went pale. I could feel the anger bubbling deep inside of her, ready to explode at any moment.

"Do you have anything to say for yourself?" she asked, her foot aggressively pushing down on the accelerator as we swiftly exited our cul-de-sac.

I sat quietly, too scared to say anything so I decided to blatantly ignore her question. My small body slumped into the seat with my hands resting in my lap. The tension in the air was thick.

Before I had any time to prepare or comprehend, I felt the sharpness of her hand slapping me so hard across the face that it left a red handprint on the side of my cheek. My whole body jolted in fright. She immediately turned to look at me with her eyes wide open, just as stunned as I was.

"Eb, I'm so sorry. I didn't mean to hit you so hard."

I continued to sit in silence, cupping my cheek in my hand to dull the sting.

* * * * *

A few weeks later, I found myself in a similar situation, but this time, I thought I'd be smart about it. When Mum got into the driver's seat, she turned around to see me sitting in the back seat of the car, looking at me with a very confused expression on her face.

"Eb, what are you doing back there? Get in the front," she said.

"No, I don't want to." I was adamant not to get between her and her uncontrollable temper. Her shoulders fell away from her ears, and she continued to stare at me with immense guilt in her eyes. She knew exactly why I had chosen to sit in the back and felt terrible about it. In that moment, she realised how frightened I was of her and her temper.

* * * * *

One day, I'd be avoiding getting slapped, and the next, Mum was like my best friend. I told her everything – good and bad - even if I knew I was going to get into trouble. I couldn't ever lie to her. She was too clever for that, or maybe I was just a bad liar. "You'll always get into less trouble if you tell the truth," she'd say.

One afternoon I was at my friend Sally's house, who lived around the corner from me. I considered her to be like my rebel friend; we were always up to mischief. Her dad was a heavy smoker, and being the curious nine-year-olds we were, we decided to give it a try. We found one of her dad's cigarette butts that he'd left on the driveway, snuck a lighter from inside, and as we were walking back towards my house, we found a quiet place to light it up and smoke what was left of it.

I watched as Sally inhaled her first puff deep into her lungs before blowing the white cloud of smoke into the air around us. It was like she knew exactly what she was doing. Meanwhile, I was having a mini panic attack on the inside, petrified of what Mum might say if she found out.

What if she smells it on me when I walk inside?

When it was my turn, I stood there hesitantly holding the butt in between my fingers, trying to be cool but having absolutely no idea what I was doing. I finally brought it up towards my lips and inhaled the smallest puff of air before coughing up the chemicals my lungs were clearly rejecting.

"Oh, that's gross!" I said immediately, handing it back for her to finish.

I went home later that afternoon. I don't think I'd ever packed an overnight bag so quickly in my life. I was in and out of the house in a flash, and Mum never suspected anything.

Thank goodness.

The next day, I walked into her room and sat on the edge of her bed, watching as she finished folding the clean clothes.

"Mum, I need to tell you something. I did something bad," I admitted, guilt written all over my face.

She finished folding the last pair of trousers and sat on the bed next to me as I proceeded to tell her my version of events from the day prior, sobbing through most of it.

"Please don't be mad at me. I hardly breathed anything in, and it was disgusting. I'm never doing it again. I'm sorry," I begged. She hadn't said a word, and I sat staring at my feet. I waited for her to yell at me for being so silly, and then, all of a sudden, she burst into laughter.

My brows furrowed as my head snapped up to look at her, totally confused.

"Oh, Eb, I'm not mad at you. We all try these things. As long as you don't make a habit of it," she joked and hugged me. I wrapped my arms around her and let out a heavy sigh, relief flooding through me.

"He who has a why to live can bear almost any reason how."

– Friedrich Nietzsche

6

It was three-thirty in the afternoon, and I was waiting patiently for my mum at the school pick-up zone. She didn't always pick me up; I would often get a lift home with either my neighbour or a friend who lived up the street from me. I preferred going home with other people, mostly because I wanted to mould myself into someone else's life for as long as possible before I had to face reality and return home.

As soon as I saw the metallic blue Toyota Corolla roll into the school car park, I stood up off the bench and walked towards the curb. I threw my school bag in the boot, and as I opened the car door, I felt an immediate change in my mood. Her cold, emotionless energy was suddenly being reflected through my own. She was wearing the same old clothes that she had put on this morning and had her sandy blonde hair tied back in a loose ponytail; I could tell she hadn't bothered to blow dry her fringe today.

"How was your day?" she asked in the same monotonous voice that had become so familiar to me.

"Good," I replied, mimicking her level of enthusiasm.

I put my seat belt on, resting my chin on my fist and looking out the window.

"What did you do today?"

"Nothing interesting," I mumbled.

"What's wrong?" she asked sharply. She was starting to lose patience.

"Nothing's wrong," I turned my head to look at her, trying to sound convincing.

Her eyes quickly narrowed, and her breath deepened in frustration.

"Why are you always like this after school?" she snapped.

"I just don't feel like talking," I replied. I had no intention to give her what she wanted.

"I'm not your slave, Ebonie, and I don't appreciate you ignoring me every time I pick you up."

I didn't know exactly why I was always so closed off and unresponsive every time she picked me up, but something about her gloomy, low-spirited presence really got on my nerves. All I wanted to do was sit in silence and watch the world pass by as we drove the rest of the way home.

* * * * *

As we got out of the car, I noticed Mum walking with a slight limp with each step she took. I looked down and realised her foot was completely black and blue and very swollen.

"Mum, what happened to your foot?" I asked, this time with a little more expression in my voice.

"I was doing some gardening today and tripped down the stairs. I'll put some ice on it after dinner. It's fine," she replied lightly.

We had a set of ten or so stairs with a garden on either side that led from our back patio down to the area of grass below.

That explains the daggy clothes today, I thought.

Later that evening, Mum was busy preparing dinner for the two of us, and I had set myself up at the dining table in front of the kitchen bench to do my homework. I turned around to ask her a question when something suddenly caught my eye. She had a deep, angry red mark that appeared to wrap around the front of her neck, just below her jawline.

"Why is your neck red?" I asked, completely disregarding my initial question.

Her eyes didn't leave the knife as she continued to chop up the vegetables.

"Oh, it's nothing. I think it's just a rash from being in the garden today."

Something wasn't sitting right, but I accepted her explanation and returned to my homework.

A few moments went by, and then the chopping suddenly stopped.

"I tried to hang myself today," she said abruptly.

I immediately let go of my pencil. My heart clenched. I turned around to face her, and looked directly into her dreary blue eyes.

"What do you mean you tried to hang yourself today? Is that why your foot is bruised?" My eyes widened in shock as everything began to piece together. I couldn't understand the words that had just come out of her mouth.

She lowered her chin towards her chest, and her eyes winced like she didn't know what to say next.

"No, it's not," she said, shaking her head, clearly distressed. "I did just trip down the stairs…"

"You wouldn't just say that, Mum! Tell me what happened," I demanded.

She paused for a moment to compose herself.

"The rope broke, and I fell. I must have landed on my ankle. I'm sorry, Eb. I shouldn't have said anything to you," her voice was full of regret.

I could feel the heat radiating from my cheeks as I continued to sit there in disbelief.

"I know this might sound strange, but when I woke up, I knew that God had spoken to me," she continued. "He sent me a message to tell me that leaving you was not the answer," her voice broke.

I stood up off the chair and walked around to hug her, both of us now crying into each other's arms. I was in such a state of shock, my brain was in overdrive, trying to process the information I had just received. But I was so relieved that she was still here. Now, all I wanted her to tell me was that she was never going to try it again.

* * * * *

After her self-inflicted, near-fatal incident, Mum was suddenly inspired to write a testimonial to share with our church community. We had recently started attending a church service that was conveniently held in my school hall every Sunday evening. Although Mum had enrolled me into a Christian school, I hadn't been baptised as a baby, and we had never been involved in any kind of religious practice. I didn't care so much about reading the Bible or learning about God, but it started to become one of my favourite nights of the week. I felt an overwhelming sense of comfort, peace and acceptance when I walked into the room. It was like everyone around me had so much love to give, and I was ready to accept it with open arms.

It was also one of the only times that my mum left the house, and I knew that she'd fake a smile, even if it were just for a few hours.

One evening, Mum wrote and shared her story with the community. She made it very clear to everyone that she was not in a good headspace but was finally ready to turn her life around, change her mindset and be the mother she wanted to be for her only child. She received a lot of love and support after this, as did I. People finally knew the truth about what she was going through – what we were both going through – outside of these walls.

It was this newfound connection that she had suddenly created with God, with some higher power, that gave her the hope that she needed and helped her to see that life was worth living and that she had so much more to live for. She had me to live for.

"It's not about living a life free of pain, heartache or struggle. It's about cultivating a deep-rooted sense of peace that extends beyond what happens day to day. It's about remembering that no storm lasts forever."

– Michell Clark

7

I was slightly nervous about being left alone with a girl who I barely knew outside of dancing while our mothers went out for a cute date night together to watch a live show, but my heart felt happy knowing Mum was leaving the house with her new friend.

I hadn't known Lucy for that long; I'd never been to her house before or spent time one-on-one with her, which made me feel a little awkward as we lay there watching Bubble Boy, a film about a boy who was born without an immune system and had to live his life in a physical bubble to protect his health. Ironically, it reminded me of how Mum lived her life.

When our parents arrived home later that evening, the first thing I noticed was a huge shift in Mum's energy. When she walked through the front door, I immediately felt the warmth of the positivity radiating from her like rays of sunshine penetrating my skin on a cool winter's morning. Her posture was tall but relaxed, with collarbones that smiled, along with the sparkle in her eyes that I knew wasn't there before. It was the happiest I'd seen her in months.

As we got into the car, I was pleasantly surprised to see her vibrant energy was not just an act; she was still oozing joy and smiling from ear to ear.

"Did you have a good time tonight, Mum?" I felt a sudden eagerness to engage in conversation, knowing she wanted to as well.

"Oh Eb, I had the best night. Rachel is such a lovely person, and I am going to try to go out with her more often," she gushed. A wave of relief swept through me, and I could tell from the excitement in her voice she was completely genuine.

Maybe this is exactly what she needs! Maybe things will be different now, I thought.

It was the glimmer of hope I needed. I looked over at her and smiled, feeling so grateful she had finally felt the pure happiness she had been longing for. I just hoped it was here to stay.

* * * * *

The next morning, I eagerly sprung out of my bed and ran across the hall into my mum's room before softly jumping up onto her bed, hoping she would mimic my enthusiasm. "Good morning!" I exclaimed.

"Morning, Bub," she replied monotonously. She seemed irritated that I'd woken her. I gently laid my head onto the pillow next to hers and felt a sudden flood of frustration weighing down my body. I knew straight away from her melancholic tone that she was not the same person that she was last night.

"Are we going to the markets today?" I asked enthusiastically, still trying to determine the level of misery this day would entail. I loved going to the farmers markets with Mum on a Sunday morning to buy our fresh, organic produce; something about it felt so soothing to me. It was an outing for us that I knew for sure wasn't going to spike her anxiety.

"Yes, I'll get up soon. Just give me a little while. Go watch some TV," she replied, clearly wanting me to leave her in peace. It felt like she wanted to stay in bed forever, twenty-four hours a day. I understood that it was her safe haven, the only place where she felt completely at ease, but I just wanted her to want to get out of bed for once. To get up, to be happy and want to live. That flicker of hope I'd had twelve hours ago had once again, very much disappeared.

"Happiness requires struggle. Without struggle, the world would lack meaning and our joys would feel empty. Be grateful for your struggles, because within them is the constant opportunity for purpose."

– Mark Manson

8

If I ever needed to escape from the gloominess of my own home, I would go play with the little girl next door. I met Jessica not long before my parents separated, before she could even talk in full sentences. Although she was four years younger than me, she became my best friend, more like my little sister, and I became a part of her family – a family that represented what I imagined a normal family to be like.

Her parents were around the same age as mine, happily married and worked mostly from home within the film production industry, designing and modelling the most intricate objects for different film sets. With their main film genre being based around science fiction, many of their models were spaceships, aircraft, robots, water vessels, and although they weren't to scale, I was always in awe of how life-like they looked without realising how much time and energy went into each design. When the work was there, the income was decent, but it wasn't always consistent, which meant that money was often quite tight, and they always had to plan ahead.

When it came to money and being able to afford nice things, Jessica and I had been brought up living a very similar lifestyle. Our concept of money was still very much in the developing stages, but our parents made it very clear that, unfortunately for us, money did not grow on trees, and we needed to earn the things we wanted. Although we never went without, contrary to the opinion of many, being a single child did not mean that we got spoilt.

Mum was quite frugal when it came to spending money, even though she didn't always need to be. Unless it was a necessity, like a school or dance uniform, I was rarely given things with the original price tag still on them. My greatest excitement was going to a charity shop to buy 'new' second-hand clothes. For my birthday or Christmas presents, if I ever wanted a big-ticket item, Mum would try her best to find a cheaper option or buy a pre-owned version. It never bothered me; sometimes, I didn't even know.

I had a weekly pocket money allowance of ten dollars. Mum would hand it to me in cash at the end of each week, but only if I had ticked off the list of household chores pinned to the fridge: unload the dishwasher, make my bed, fold and put away my clean clothes, pull the large rubbish bins up to the top of our steep driveway on a Sunday evening ready for rubbish collection on Monday morning. I earned even extra if I mowed the lawns or washed the car.

It became a learnt behaviour not to spend my pocket money on trivial items like toys, lollies, or things I knew I wouldn't use. Unless it was something I really wanted, I held onto this money like I was never going to see any more. My mum taught me to be practical, purposeful, and sensible with my dollars, a skill she knew would set me up for life.

My everlasting enthusiasm for going to a market began when I was about eight years old when Jessica's mum would take us to a local car boot sale almost every weekend. There was something so thrilling to me about waking up at the crack of dawn, ten minutes before I had to rush next door so we could get to the market early enough to find the best deals. I loved meandering my way through the rows of pop-up stalls, sifting through the things that people were selling for a fraction of the price they initially bought them for. I became an expert bargain hunter, and it soon became my favourite day of the week.

Jessica's home became a safe space for me; somewhere I went when I felt I had nowhere else to go. Her home was somewhere I could be a kid and do normal kid things without ridiculous restrictions, and no one could be disappointed in me if I accidentally moved something out of place or left my colouring pencils out on the table after I'd finished using them. I got to experience a sense of normality that I just didn't have otherwise.

* * * * *

Decorating the Christmas tree was one of my favourite jobs of the year, and as soon as I became old enough, my mum was glad to let me do it all by myself. We had a standard store-bought medium-sized green tree that I decorated with baubles of all different shapes, colours and sizes, some of which I'd made in kindergarten. I'd then wrap the tree with red, gold and silver tinsel, whatever we had really, starting from the top and making my way to the bottom before finishing with the multi-coloured string lights, which, in my opinion, were the most tedious part of the job. I always felt they added no value to the aesthetic until the sun had gone down, and even then, we'd forget to turn them on. The tree ended up looking like a rainbow had spat it out, with no obvious order or colour scheme.

Christmas morning had rolled around yet again, and I was up bright and early, ready and raring to finally be able to rip into the presents that had been sitting under the tree for weeks. I never expected to get a lot for Christmas, but it didn't stop me from getting excited about the few presents I did get.

Christmas morning had always been the three of us, but after Dad moved out and Mum became the way she was, the whole thing became a little less enjoyable. Although she tried, it was obvious she never shared the same level of enthusiasm for Christmas as I did. It was just another day to her, another day to sit in misery and hibernate in the comfort of her own home. She didn't want to socialise with anyone or share the day with other people, she was content being alone.

She managed to get herself out of bed with a little bit of encouragement from me and met me in the lounge room where I was sitting on the mat in front of the tree, waiting patiently for her engagement. She sat down on the couch, holding her hot cup of herbal tea, and watched as I began making my way through the presents with my name on them.

A gentle smile lit up across her face as I handed her the small gift that I had bought for her at one of my recent trips to the markets, as well as the card I had made for her with the bits and bobs from my craft box. Designing a card or some kind of gift for my close friends and family was something I thoroughly enjoyed doing. I grew to see it as an opportunity to express my gratitude for the person in a way that was more sentimental and sincere. Whether it be for her birthday, Mother's Day or Christmas, my mum's card would always include some form of apology for all the things I had done wrong, with the intention of showing her that I was trying to be a better child.

The last present I had to unwrap was one that my mum had shown the most excitement for the entire morning. I quickly tore through the wrapping paper and pulled out a brand-new, rather expensive looking, delicately crocheted blue cardigan with a cutout shape of a butterfly on the back. My shoulders immediately dropped in disappointment as I held the rather expensive piece of clothing up in front of me. I didn't know what I was expecting, but I wished it was something else.

"Don't you like it?" she asked, her tone saddened and her eyes darkened.

"Yeah," I replied bluntly as I put the cardigan down next to the rest of my presents beside me.

"Well, a thank you would be nice," she snapped, realising I had shown no appreciation for the thought she had put into my gift.

"Thank you," I mumbled forcefully. "Can I please go to Jessica's now?"

"You only care about the presents," she stood up from the couch in frustration and headed towards the kitchen to wash up her mug.

"No, I don't, Mum! I'm sorry, but they said they'd wait until I got there to start opening their presents," I argued back, trying to hide the real reason as to why I wanted to leave. After having spent the last few Christmases with Jessica and her family, it had now become our little tradition – I no longer had to be invited; they just automatically assumed that I would be there.

"Yep, fine. Go," she waved her hand at me as if to say 'I don't care, just leave me alone.'

I grabbed my things, put my shoes on and walked out the front door.

A pit of guilt sat deep in my stomach and only began to grow rapidly. I don't know what had come over me. I had been so ungrateful, and I felt terrible for it. As I walked towards Jessica's front door, I continued to replay the scene over and over in my head. Every part of me wished I could cut and retake that part of my morning out so I could react differently, even if I had to force myself to pretend a little. I felt like I had completely destroyed any sparkle of joy Mum had been willing to show that morning, and it would be on my conscience for the rest of the day.

* * * * * *

I'd arrived home from spending the day next door, and we were sitting in the lounge room watching a replay of our favourite television show, Home and Away. Mum sat to the left of me, cross-legged on her single-seated soft brown recliner chair, and I was sat on mine with my fluffy red blanket covering my outstretched legs.

Mum would always mute the ad breaks because she couldn't stand listening to the same repetitive crap over and over. After a few seconds, she suddenly broke the silence.

"If anything were to happen to me, would you want to live with your dad or with Aunty Jan?" She looked at me as if this was a completely normal question to ask your ten-year-old daughter on a regular weeknight. I sat for a moment, pondering her very random query.

"I'd want to live with Aunty Jan," I answered after a few seconds. It wasn't a hard decision for me to make; I knew that living with my dad would hardly be an option. "Why?" I questioned her.

"I thought you might have said that. I'm just making some changes to my Will, and this is something I need to include," she said.

She turned her head back towards the television and pressed the unmute button just as Home and Away returned to the screen. Nothing more was said.

"If you focus on protecting your heart, you can avoid a lot of pain. But you can also end up living half a life."

– Virgin River

9

It had been about five years since my parents separated when Mum decided she wanted to enter the dating world again. Technology had notably evolved by this time, which meant the newspaper days were over, and she was able to set up a profile on an online dating site, eHarmony.

Age: 49 | *Height:* 5' 9" | *Ethnicity:* White, Australian

Occupation: Sales representative | *Education:* Bachelor's degree

Smoking: Never | *Drinking:* Never

Kids: a ten-year-old daughter

Interests & Hobbies: Music, Movies, Walking, Beach, Baking

I am most passionate about:

Loving myself and those around me, especially my daughter. Staying fit and healthy. Eating well and living a natural, organic lifestyle.

How I typically spend my leisure time:
I enjoy spending time outdoors, going for walks along the beach,
watching movies or reading a good book.

What I am looking for:
I am looking for someone to share quality time and do fun things with
on the weekends. Someone who will accept both my daughter
and me.

It didn't take long for my mum's profile to be noticed by several potential matches. There was one that instantly took her fancy: Chris. He was a few years older than Mum and had two older children of his own who had already moved out of home. He worked as an electrician, which meant that he had to be somewhat intellectual and physically fit. It was obvious from his profile photos that he was tall and slim in stature and had very kind brown eyes behind his rectangle-shaped glasses. He was a non-smoker, didn't drink and appeared to have the same interests as my mum – on paper, they were the perfect match.

They formed a very special connection right from the beginning, and my mum knew he was everything she was looking for. He was laid back, gentle and very considerate towards her needs – he understood I was her top priority and anyone who came into her life would have to be accepting of that. Chris quickly fell head over heels for my mum and was willing to do anything to make her happy, but he wanted things to move a lot faster than what she was ready for, or maybe faster than what I was prepared for. I had already met him a handful of times when he came over one night for dinner. He was always so lovely towards me and had never done anything to make me think otherwise, but it didn't stop me from not wanting him around.

I reluctantly greeted him with a forced smile on my face as he walked through our front door. The unpleasant knots in my stomach tightened some more as I watched him give my mum and quick peck on the lips before following her into the dining room to take a seat. He continued to engage in conversation with my mum, trying his best to include me as well, but I didn't want a bar of it. I could see how hard he was trying, and every part of my heart wanted to feel okay about it. I wanted to like the man that my mum was clearly so happy with. But whenever there was any form of physical affection between him and my mum, a wave of intense emotion washed over me – jealousy, fear, anger – feelings that quickly manifested into a nasty attitude that took complete control over my behaviour.

I walked into the darkness of my bedroom, curled myself up under the blankets on my bed and buried my head into my pillow while the sickening pit in my stomach grew bigger. After a few minutes of wallowing in my self-pity, I noticed my room suddenly start to get a little brighter as my mum opened my bedroom door to check on me.

"Eb, what's wrong?" she asked, coming to sit on the edge of my bed and resting her hand gently on my shoulder. I burst into tears.

"I'm sorry, Mum, I can't help it," I cried. I couldn't understand why I was feeling or acting the way I was.

Why couldn't I just be happy she had met a nice person to spend time with? Why did I envy him so much before I'd even given him a chance?

"Eb, Chris is trying to get to know you. I want you to be okay with him being here; otherwise, he will go," she sighed.

I didn't know what to say. I lay there quietly with my head tucked under the covers, just wanting to disappear completely. I could see how torn she was. Once again, I was the problem. I saw this man as an intruder, someone who was going to take my mum away from me, but this was never his intention at all.

I tried to learn how to accept this new man into our lives. I tried to be okay with my mum giving her love and affection to someone else, but I couldn't control the physical ache that lingered in the bottom of my stomach. Whenever they would spend time together, a tight feeling would wrap around my heart, or I would behave possessively with Mum whenever he was around.

After about six months, my mum decided to call it off with Chris, but it wasn't because of me. Although my mum really liked him, there was always a part of her that was afraid to be vulnerable, unable to surrender and let him in completely. I don't think she knew why, and she tried her hardest to work through it, to take things slow and ease into a new relationship, but her fears were too strong, and she struggled to overcome them.

A short time after Mum broke up with Chris, I found myself lying next to her in bed one morning, and the conversation moved to Dad. The bond that Mum and I shared was like no other connection I had in my life. I knew that she would always tell me the truth, even if sometimes it was probably a better idea to keep it to herself.

A memory had popped into my head that I just couldn't shake. When I was about four or five years old, towards the end of each week, my dad would go out for work dinner or drinks with his other colleagues.

'Can I please come with you tonight?' I'd beg as I jumped up and down in front of him to show my enthusiasm. I always envisioned these nights as being full of fun, laughter and, of course, an opportunity to eat my favourite thick-cut fries.

'Not tonight, Bub, but I'll take you out for dinner another time,' he'd say. He'd try to let me down easily, but it was the same answer every single time. He'd get home so late that I'd be in my bed, asleep already, upset that I'd missed out on hugging him goodnight. Some days, he wouldn't get back until the next morning, so I assumed that he must have stayed at a friend's place overnight.

I began to question Mum about those nights that Dad would tell me he was going out for a work event. I couldn't shake this awful feeling that he hadn't been totally honest with me, and I wanted confirmation.

"I'm sorry, Eb, but he never went out with work friends," she said. "He went to see Mandy."

I quickly propped myself up onto one arm and looked directly into Mum's eyes with my mouth wide open in shock. I had met Mandy out for dinner a handful of times soon after my parents split, and my dad moved out once he clearly didn't have to keep her a secret anymore. She was a very quiet and reserved lady, who I thought was nice but a little difficult to talk to.

"So, he was lying to me the whole time? Did you know about it?" My brain was ticking over a hundred miles an hour, struggling to understand how my parents were living in the same house, still together, as far as I knew, and yet my dad was actually seeing another woman!

"Yes, I knew about it the whole time. It was something we had discussed," she said. I couldn't believe it. She was so calm like it had never bothered her at all.

"But you were still together!" I exclaimed, still trying to understand.

"We wanted to stay living together so you had a stable home, but we agreed that we were no longer together," she explained.

"You didn't have to do that for me, Mum," I said to her, immediately feeling bad that they had tried to maintain this because of me. She looked at me with sincere appreciation in her eyes as if to say 'thank you'.

"I can't believe that but it kind of makes a little more sense now. Thank you for telling me the truth," I said softly as I wiggled myself closer towards her and gently placed my arm over her chest.

*"Keep your face to the sun and
you will never see the shadows."*

– Helen Keller

10

Like most young children, I went through a prolonged but unsuccessful phase of trying to convince Mum it was a good idea for us to get a puppy. Her classic response was always the same: "No Eb, I know I'll end up being the one taking full responsibility for it, and I don't have the time nor do I want to do that."

"No, you won't, Mum; I promise I'll look after it!" I'd say. "I'll take it for walks, feed it, bathe it. You won't have to do anything!" My twelve-year-old brain was too naive to consider the ongoing cost involved in owning a dog. It didn't matter what I said or how hard I tried; to my disappointment, her answer was always a solid no.

One morning she walked into my room to tell me she had found a breeder located in Brisbane who had a litter of boxer puppies for sale. I nearly fell over!

"I've done some research on different dog breeds, and boxers appear to be one of the most intelligent but playful dogs," she said. "They don't bark a lot and are easy to take care of."

Is she feeling okay? I wondered.

I stood up from my desk chair to face her, my cheeks beaming with excitement.

"Does that mean we are getting a dog?" I didn't care what type of dog it was; I just wanted a little friend by my side.

"Well, if we do, I'd like to get a female," she said. "And there is only one girl puppy left for sale that the lady said we can visit next week. She will be eight weeks old by then, which means she will be ready to go to a new home."

It wasn't a straight yes, but it was certainly looking to be that way.

"Thank you, thank you, thank you!" I shrieked, jumping up and down before wrapping my arms around her waist.

"What should we call her?" I instantly began to brainstorm potential names that I liked. "Mia, Ruby, Izzy... Bella?"

"Whatever you like, Bub, she'll be your puppy, but I do like Bella," Mum replied.

Bella, it is, I thought.

*****

When we arrived at the breeder's house and walked inside, we were immediately greeted by the three remaining tiny boxer puppies trotting around amongst our feet.

"Hello, come through!" the lady called, motioning us into her lounge room where the pup's mother lay splayed out on her side with her large, swollen teats fully exposed.

"This one will be yours," she said, pointing towards a puppy I'd hoped would be mine from the moment I stepped through the front door. She was different and unique in her appearance, and I liked that.

I crouched down to gently stroke her soft, shiny, fawn-coloured coat, and when her dark brown eyes met mine, I was able to admire her pitch-black snout that was marked with a very thin white stripe running down her nose. She lifted her paw, which looked like it had been dipped into white paint, up onto my hand, and I felt an immediate connection with her.

"We decided to name her Bella, but please feel free to change it to whatever you like."

I froze for a brief second. I couldn't believe my ears. "That's exactly what we were going to call her!" I exclaimed. At that moment, I knew she was meant to be mine.

* * * * *

"Now there will be rules about her being in the house," Mum warned, looking at me through the review mirror so she knew she had my attention. I sat in the back seat with Bella curled up in her temporary transport bed, comforting her on our drive home.

"She will be an outside dog during the day, but I'll allow her to come inside at night time so long as she sits on her mat in the lounge room," she continued. "She won't be allowed on the furniture, and we will need to toilet train her so she doesn't have any accidents inside."

"Can I cuddle her on the couch if she's wrapped in a blanket?" I asked, already starting to test the boundaries.

"We'll see," she replied tentatively.

I knew that getting a dog was a big thing for Mum. I think it made her even more anxious than she already was, but she did it for me because she knew it would make me happy and give me a sense of responsibility that she couldn't necessarily teach me herself.

"Thank you, Mum. I love her so much already." I couldn't wipe the smile off my face.

"You always have a choice. To remain as you are in the place that you are or to grow, to evolve. The way you choose to see the world will create the world you begin to see. Each and every day is an opportunity to choose how you are going to see it."

– Nikki Dyer

11

She began walking through a dark, eerie cave that had no exit in sight. The deeper she went, the faster the light behind her started to fade until she reached a point of complete darkness. She was lost, unsure of which direction she needed to turn to find the right path again. Her body ached and shivered as she sat there all alone. She became so exhausted, so malnourished and frail, that she eventually gave up on trying to find a way out.

Every day I thought to myself, maybe she'll wake up a little brighter. Perhaps today will be different. I prayed for a happy, healthy mum who was excited by the prosperity of life – some days, my prayers would come true. Other days, it was clear they hadn't even been heard.

I had been spending a lot of my time next door playing with Jessica during the last couple of weeks of school holidays, which were sadly coming to an end. It was nine o'clock on a Thursday morning, and I had quickly popped home to ask Mum for some money for the indoor rock climbing centre we were going to. She walked into the kitchen for the first time that morning to see me rummaging through her purse. I didn't even have to look at her to feel the sadness radiating from her body, zapping any hope I had for that day, and I instantly felt frustrated with her for no apparent reason.

I looked up at her with pleading eyes. It appeared to make no difference to her demeanour.

"Mum, why are you always so unhappy? It's like you're not even trying to get better."

She bent down to grab a mug out of the bottom cupboard before standing back up to look back at me. Her weary eyes seemed to struggle at the thought of getting through another day.

"Ebonie, please don't say that. You know I am trying as hard as I can."

I was so sick of hearing this response.

"Well, you're not trying hard enough!" I yelled back at her. I just wanted to get out of there.

"I'm going rock climbing with Jessica. Can I please have some money?"

She grabbed her purse and willingly handed me the cash I needed with no further questions, almost like she was glad to have me out of her hair.

"Thanks," I said bluntly and stormed out of the house without saying another word.

* * * * *

I sat quietly in the back seat of the car, staring out the window, wishing I could take back what I had said to Mum, but my apology would have to wait until I got home.

It was my first time indoor rock climbing, and while I was enjoying the distraction, I was on edge. I had a sudden urge to call Mum to say sorry for the way I spoke to her and to make sure she was okay. But this meant that I would have to ask Jessica's mum to borrow her phone, and I didn't want to make a big deal out of what I kept telling myself was nothing. I tried my best to ignore the heavy pit of guilt sitting at the bottom of my stomach. I'd be home soon.

A couple of hours later, we pulled into the driveway.

"I'm just going to go home quickly to grab something, and then I'll be back," I told Jessica in a rush. I couldn't shake this awful, anxious feeling; something just felt terribly wrong. I raced home, frantically opened the front door and removed my shoes so that I wouldn't get into more trouble. I ran down the narrow hallway, passing through the kitchen on my right, until I got to the dining room table that sat in front of the sliding door to the back patio. I let out a huge sigh of relief when I saw my mum standing outside, looking down at Bella, wandering around at her feet. But before any words could leave my mouth, I felt the air instantly rush from my lungs. An enormous wave of nausea washed over me, causing my knees to buckle beneath me. My heart felt like it had stopped beating, but in the same moment, my chest felt like it was going to explode.

"No, no, no," I cried as I ripped open the fly screen door and ran towards her, wrapping my arms tightly around her waist. I took one look up at her pale face and immediately pulled away. I began to scream. Uncontrollably scream.

Jessica and her mother heard my wailing from inside their house.

Instinctively, they raced over as fast as they could and found me around the corner, collapsing to the ground, struggling to take my next breath.

"Ebonie, what's wrong? What happened?" Clare asked me desperately. I trembled as I tried to stand back up. I looked over in their direction, my eyes full of complete shock and horror.

"She's... dead."

They swung open the back gate and ran towards me, and before they had any time to prepare themselves for what was coming, they saw her lifeless body hanging from the patio ceiling.

* * * * *

The next thing I knew, I was on the phone with a lady from the emergency line, pacing up and down my neighbour's living room, having what felt like some sort of panic attack.

"Are you still there, Ebonie?" the lady continued to repeat over and over, ensuring I remained on the phone with her.

"Yes, I'm here. Please help her," I begged. "I need to do something to help her. I don't know what to do. What do I do?" I was full of fear and uncertainty.

"You just need to stay on the phone with me right where you are and wait until the ambulance arrives. They will help her," she said, trying her best to comfort me.

I wanted to trust her, but what did she know? She hadn't seen what I saw. All I kept saying was, "What if it's too late? What if they can't help her?"

I was in denial. I didn't want to believe what I had seen, but the day just kept unravelling in ways I struggled to accept.

My other neighbour was now sitting next to me as I sat on the edge of the couch, staring blankly into space, rocking my body anxiously back and forth. Suddenly, I broke the silence with a question I had been petrified to ask but needed to know the answer to.

"Is she really dead?" I finally brought myself to say.

She looked at me and paused for a few moments as she mustered up the will to confess quite possibly one of the hardest things that she would ever have to tell a twelve-year-old child. I knew then what her response was going to be, but I hoped with every inch of my being I was wrong.

"I'm so sorry, Ebonie. Yes, she is gone."

In that moment, I crumbled. This time, it was all too real.

* * * * *

I used my neighbour's phone to call the two people who I needed most – Aunty Jan, who was in Melbourne visiting her family, and then Dad.

"Hello, Jan speaking," Aunty Jan answered the unknown number brightly. She sounded a million miles away.

"Aunty Jan, it's me, Ebonie," I said, trying to hold back my tears for a least the first sentence.

"Ebonie, hi! Is everything okay?"

She could hear the tremble in my voice but also knew that something must have been wrong for me to be calling on someone else's phone.

"No. Um… it's Mum," I said, trying to find the words. "She's… She's dead."

I crumbled.

"Oh, Ebonie, what happened? Where are you?" The questions began to roll off her tongue.

"I'm at Jessica's house, and the ambulance is there with her. I don't know what to do," I replied, feeling a wave of panic shoot through me all over again.

"I'll book the next flight home and be there as soon as I can, Ebonie. Please call me if you need anything. I'm coming. I love you," she said. For the calmest person I knew, she sounded the most distraught I'd ever heard her.

* * * * *

I swiftly got up from the same spot on the couch I'd been sitting on all afternoon and walked towards the front door after hearing the doorbell ring. My eyes widened with whatever joy I had when I saw Dad standing behind the screen door, waiting to be let in. I pulled down on the handle to let him in, and any form of happiness I was feeling instantly disappeared the moment I saw his girlfriend hiding behind him.

I pretended I was delighted to see her as a wave of anger simultaneously washed over me.

Why did he have to bring her?

He sat next to me on the couch and gently wrapped one arm around my shoulders while his other hand held hers. I watched as they looked into each other's eyes, jealousy sinking into my bones. I wanted to be sick. My mother had just died, and it still wasn't enough for me to be the centre of my father's world. My heart had been shattered, and, at that moment, I knew I could no longer rely on him to pick up the pieces.

"Do you want a slice of pizza?" he asked, pointing towards the takeaway pizza box that was sitting on the coffee table in front of us.

"No thanks. I'm not hungry."

I sat in silence, staring blankly into the distance while conversations happening around me slowly faded into the background. My brain was trying to filter through the flood of thoughts circulating my mind at a million miles an hour before stumbling on a question I couldn't find an answer to.

How is it possible for me to feel so alone in a room full of people? To miss someone so deeply and crave their attention so badly when they are sitting right next to me?

Physically, my dad was there, but he may as well not have been.

* * * * *

I was lying in my neighbour's spare bed, trying to fall asleep. Every time I closed my eyes, I saw the heart-wrenching visions of my mother's unconscious face, something I knew I'd never be able to un-see. I quickly opened my eyes, hoping to remove the unwanted images from my mind. I laid on my back as still as a plank of wood, looking up at the ceiling, scared to the bone of how I was going to live without her.

I woke the next morning, my eyes still red and puffy. My stomach felt like it was tied up in thousands of mini knots. I wasn't sure if I wanted to vomit or if I was just really hungry. I didn't think it would be possible for me to feel even more numb than I had the day before, but I did.

"Did my mum leave me a note or anything?" I asked Clare, hoping she had found something that I had missed.

"Yes, she did. I was going to wait to give it to you, but I'll get it for you now."

She handed me the single piece of paper that Mum had left for me.

"There were some drops of water on the top of the page when I found it. I'm assuming they were her tears."

"Thank you," I took the page from her hands and went to my room to read it.

I am sorry, Ebonie,
I just can't go on in this torment.
It is not your fault – please don't blame yourself.
I love you – I'm just a tormented soul, and I need to put it to rest.
Ring Aunty Jan and she will help sort things out for you.
Please forgive me.
Love Mum xxx

That's all? I held the letter in my hands, desperately wanting more. I wanted to know every detail of what was going through her head. It was too brief like she was in a rush to get it done.

My mum was always a big writer; it's how she expressed herself the most. She would write letters to everyone she loved and put so much thought, love and passion into her words.

Although she told me not to, I did blame myself. I knew I had been the only constant in her life for such a long time; I struggled to see how I wasn't the problem.

If I tried harder and did more for her, I thought. If I hadn't been so difficult or rude to her, maybe she'd still be here. If only I was a better child.

* * * * *

Two weeks after she died, I found a small floral notebook someone had recently gifted to me. I began writing to my mum as if I were having a conversation with her. It was the only thing that helped me to feel connected to her in some way.

13/10/2011

To my dearest mummy,

Today I went to the movies with my friend and saw Spy Kids.

I loved it!

Did you see my Naplan test results? I know you would've been impressed.

I don't know what I'm going to do without you. Why did you do that?

I miss you so much! I can't stop thinking about what happened.

Please help me, Mum.

Help me to forget it and wipe it out of my mind.

I'll always miss you.

I love you so much, and I will never forget you.

I'll talk to you tomorrow.

Lots of love always, Eb xxx

"You can shed tears that they are gone, or you can smile because they lived. You can close your eyes and pray that they will come back, or you can open your eyes and see all that they left."

– David Harkins

12

I didn't know what to expect when I walked into the small, brightly lit room where my mum lay peacefully in her coffin bed. I had been told that a viewing would give me the opportunity to say a proper goodbye, to see my mum in a state of rest, and hopefully mask the final visions I had of her.

Grief flashed through my eyes as I stood under the wooden door frame, looking in from afar. I could see my mum's hands resting delicately on her stomach, one on top of the other. I timidly stepped towards the coffin, with Jessica and her mother following closely behind me so I wasn't alone, and I noticed that she had been elegantly dressed in some of her clothes. She was wearing a pair of her navy wide legged trousers, with a white three-quarter sleeve blouse and one of her tribal beige coloured, thick beaded necklaces that she wore often. The mortician had styled her sandy blonde hair nicely so that it rested softly on her shoulders, but her makeup was heavy, more than she would've liked. It looked like my mum, but at the same time, it didn't.

I wanted to reach in and hold her hand one last time, to tell her how much I missed her and wanted her back. I slowly reached my hand inside her coffin, and when I touched her hand with my index finger, her skin was cold. Ice cold. I quickly pulled my hand away, in shock from the unexpected sensation. I felt as if the room was closing in on me. I didn't want to look at her anymore, and I didn't want to speak to her; I just wanted to get the hell out of there.

*****

I stood at the front of the hall, wearing the sky-blue crocheted cardigan that my mum had bought me last Christmas, blankly greeting everyone as they walked into the church for my mother's funeral. Family members, distant relatives, friends of my mum that I hardly recognised, and many of my friends came to show their support and give their condolences – even my school principal and a few of my teachers made a surprise appearance.

I sat on the wooden bench up towards the front of the church, resting my head on the shoulder of a close family friend who I'd met at our church, listening to the eulogy that the minister was delivering as he accurately described the story of Mum's short life.

'In tribute to Jan Robyn Stirling, who was born in Melbourne, Victoria, in February of 1960, three years after her brother Stephen. She was a child of a lot of sass and enjoyed being the centre of attention amongst her family of four.

Jan achieved high marks all through her schooling – she was an all-rounder and very good at sports, including netball and tennis, her favourite being Aussie rules footy; she wasn't afraid to run around with the boys and barge her way into a solid tackle.

After year twelve, Jan went straight on to Teachers College, where she found her passion for teaching and soon became a very talented and dedicated educator. The bonds she formed with her students were very special to her, and she realised that she had this innate ability to turn even the most troublesome students around simply by meeting them on their level and allowing them to be themselves.

When Jan moved to the Gold Coast in the early 1990s, she decided to take a break from the demands that came with being a high-school teacher and dabbled in a couple of hospitality jobs before returning to her passion once more.

It wasn't long after this when Jan met her future husband, Jason. They married in 1998, just before Jan's mother, Laurel, sadly passed away from breast cancer, which was also a few months before Ebonie was born. The passing of her mother was a very difficult time for Jan; they shared a very deep and loving bond, one that could never be replaced.

Jan managed to successfully balance being a full-time mum and a part-time teacher for the first few years after Ebonie was born before deciding to permanently leave this role behind and become a Maths Advisor and then a sales representative at a well-known education publishing company. She excelled in every role she worked in and built some special relationships along the way.

Jan was a very confident, vibrant and outgoing young woman who was often described as being 'the life of the party' by her beloved friends. She was known to be a perfectionist, an intelligent, successful and highly motivated woman who achieved anything she put her mind to. Her infectious laugh would light up any room she walked into, along with her kind, loving nature that people were so easily drawn to. This is how Jan would have wanted people to remember her.'

I realised that I had not yet shed a single tear throughout the entire service, and I didn't know why I wasn't crying.

Is there something wrong with me?

I was almost trying to force it so that people wouldn't think I was completely heartless, but I just couldn't.

When it was Aunty Jan's turn to share her story, she stood up at the altar with a couple of scrunched-up tissues in her hand, took a deep breath in and looked out to the room full of people in front of her.

'Jan was a very dear friend of mine for almost twenty years. We met not long after she moved to the Gold Coast at the Steak House pub in Surfers Paradise, where we both worked. I remember Jan only lasted three weeks in the place before quitting – she told me that she couldn't handle all the rules. But within that short time, we had managed to build a friendship that continued to flourish over many wonderful years.

Although our personalities were very different, we found comfort in the fact that we shared fairly similar upbringings; both being raised with a brother by our sides in the Southeastern suburbs of Melbourne, in a loving and relatively stable household, before deciding to take the leap and venture out to sunny Queensland.

We were both single at the time and never turned down the opportunity to hit the clubs and have a boogie. But Jan was always very popular with the boys, which meant that on almost every occasion, she'd be quickly snatched up by someone new, leaving my friend and I to our own devices while she dazzled in the limelight and danced the night away. We weren't jealous at all...' she joked. Everyone giggled.

"I was going out with my husband Rex around the same time that Jan met Jason, so we'd often go on double dates together and luckily for us, the friendship between the boys also grew.

Jan thrived throughout her pregnancy with Ebonie – it was the healthiest I'd ever seen her, and she made an incredible mother.

My friendship with Jan was filled with love and support and in the early days, so much fun and adventure. She was always the leader, the instigator and the one with all the confidence – she always took control, and I was the one who went along with the plan. But over the years, our relationship began to change drastically. After her separation from Jason, her mindset was completely different; she was exhausted all the time, and every day was becoming a greater effort. My friend was starting to slip away, and I didn't know how to bring her back," she paused, trying her best to hold back the tears. She closed her eyes and took another deep breath in before continuing.

"Although it started to become a very one-sided friendship, I chose to accept that at that moment. My friend needed my support; she needed me to be strong for her, and I was determined to stick it out. I had to do this for Ebonie. I had to make sure she was okay, and I had to give her the hope and love she deserved," her tears were now flowing, and she was struggling to get through the last few words of her speech.

"I know in my heart that I helped her through many rough times, and I feel that I was always there for her when she needed me. In the end, Jan chose her path and reached her destination, a place where she could find peace. Rest easy, my dear Jan. I promise I won't let you down."

I could feel the sadness vibrating through the room. She folded her pieces of paper and made her way back to her seat.

My mum's brother and a few others then had the opportunity to share their stories about my mum, admire her strengths and praise her achievements. At the end of the service, we watched my mum's life play through a slide show of photos with her favourite song playing in the background, 'Amazing Grace'.

The words of this song spoke to me as if my mum was telling the story right in front of me. It was then that I fell apart, and the tears began to pour down my cheeks.

"It is human nature to strive to work everything out and try to control life. But trying to make sense of every part of your life is like trying to piece together a jigsaw puzzle while having only a few small pieces of the puzzle in your possession."

– Toni Carmine Salerno

13

My mum grew up always trying to impress her father, constantly trying to be the best at everything she did, hoping to prove to him that she deserved a place on the pedestal he placed her on. The immense pressure that she put on herself not to be a failure or a disappointment, only contributed to the development of her highly strung personality.

My mum's father was extremely domineering; he was the man of the house, and everyone had to abide by his overly strict rules, including his wife, no questions asked. Mum hated the way her mum was treated, the way that he spoke to her and demanded things from her, but nothing was ever said or done about it, it was simply swept under the rug, and became a very normal part of life.

Along with his obnoxious attitude came a serious temper, one that got even worse under the influence of alcohol. He would come home after a night out at the pub, barge into my mum's room, yelling and screaming at her for no apparent reason. She would tuck herself deep under the covers, terrified of him, trying to ignore it as best as she could.

* * * * *

As I was going through my mum's more personal items, I came across a page that she had written during one of her emotional detoxes with her naturopath.

My guilt relates to Ebonie – it's almost like I feel her emotions more than she does. I feel guilty about her abandonment. She's scared but she gets on with life, but I feel the daily torment of it all.
I feel responsible for almost every aspect of her life.
I worry about her homework, her involvement in things, and I don't just let her be.
It takes all my conscious effort to let her be in control of her.
I find it hard to be a mother and just guide her without taking on the worries of her life.
That's what has been overwhelming me.
I need to hand over the guilt to God and allow Ebonie to just be who she is.

My mum was a perfectionist in many ways and always put an unbelievable amount of pressure on herself to be the best in all aspects of her life, a quality of hers that I truly admired. But with that came a compelling need to be in control, not only over her life but mine, too. When it came to my schooling and education, she took great pride in me being a top student, so much so that she would start helping me with my school projects and assignments only to end up completely taking over and essentially doing them for me.

She sat with me for hours, making up flashcards, listening to me rehearse my English speeches over and over, or helping me to memorise my times tables, and we wouldn't stop until I got it right. In her mind, failing simply wasn't an option.

She struggled to let me do things for myself without her input, to make my own mistakes and then learn how to do better next time. Much like her father had done for her, she set incredibly high standards for me to achieve the best results, or be the best at everything I did, and if I failed in some way, it would be like she had failed too. It came from the goodness of her heart but to the detriment of her mental well-being. The burden she held became too much, and it began to eat at her from the inside out.

* * * * *

I wasn't sure how I felt about the entire seventh grade knowing about my mother's passing when I returned to school a week after everything happened. They didn't know how, only that she had 'passed away tragically.'

I wanted to hide under an invisibility cloak as I walked into class, holding my heavy textbooks in my arms. I sat down at my desk and pulled out my English book in preparation for my first class. I stared down at the words on the page in front of me and suddenly felt a paralysing anxiety cave in on top of me.

How am I going to manage this all by myself? How am I going to keep getting good grades without Mum here to help me? What if I don't understand any of it and I fail? Tears began to fill my eyes at the thought of being so alone. I had always been a goody two shoes - always in the running for an academic award or some other recognition. I was disappointed if I got anything below straight As, but I had zero confidence in myself to get the same grades on my own without Mum's help. None of it came naturally to me, and I was terrified of letting her down. I couldn't stand the thought of being a failure.

"Forgiveness is accepting the apology
you will never receive."

– Shawne Duperon

14

My neighbour gently pulled open the sliding glass door of my new psychologist's office and stepped to the side, allowing me to walk on in front of her. The receptionist looked up from her computer, smiled cheerfully at me and generously welcomed us inside. She directed us to take a seat on one of the three cushioned black chairs up against the wall of the waiting area, and I sat nervously on the edge of my seat, staring down at my knees as they jittered up and down.

It had been six weeks since the passing of my mum, and still, nothing about my life felt real. I was completely numb, unsure of how I was going to survive without her.

I suddenly heard footsteps coming from the small corridor around the corner, forcing me to break my gaze from the floor and direct my attention to the very tall, broad-shouldered lady now standing in front of me. Her gorgeously thick, curly blonde hair dangled just above her shoulders as she looked down at me with her kind blue eyes and welcomed me in the direction of her office. My neighbour and I followed behind her as she showed us to her room.

When I walked through the door, I noticed three large black leather chairs situated in the shape of a triangle with a patterned rug in the centre. I sat down on the chair opposite Shannon and tried my best to avoid any eye contact with her for as long as possible. I sat with my hands tucked under my bottom, my shoulders shrugged up towards my ears and continued to trace my eyes along the pattern of the rug. My body was completely frozen, and I didn't know what I was supposed to say. I struggled to find the words to describe how I was feeling, fearful of reliving the experience all over again. I just wanted to shut myself off from the world around me and forget it all. Or better yet, wake up from the nightmare I so desperately hoped it was.

* * * * *

I had been seeing Shannon once a week for a month, trying to work through the immense hurt and sadness I was feeling. It was our fifth session together, and I had a burning question I almost felt too guilty to ask. I held my hands together, fiddling around with my fingers and continued to stare down at Shannon's feet.

"Is it okay for me to feel kind of relieved now that my mum is gone?" I looked at her with shame in my eyes and continued.

"I feel really bad for saying this, but it almost feels like my life is a little better now." The moment the words left my mouth, it felt like I had completely betrayed my mum.

"She always told me how my life would be better off without her, and of course, I told her it wasn't true… but maybe in some ways, she was right?"

Admitting this to myself and speaking the words aloud made me feel instant relief, like a weight had been lifted off my shoulders. Shannon took a moment before answering my question.

"Ebonie, feeling a sense of relief is completely natural. Your mum wasn't a happy person, and she put you through a lot at such a young age. Now you are free from always worrying about her, and you know she is finally at peace within herself."

I felt a sudden shift in my energy. I didn't feel like such a terrible daughter anymore because I knew that what I was feeling was completely valid. Obviously, I wish things were different. I would've done anything to bring my mum back, but maybe there was a silver lining beneath all the heartache. I was very glad to have finally gotten that off my chest.

* * * * *

As the shock of it all began to settle and I moved past the point of denial, I began to realise how incredibly angry I was at my mum. She had turned my entire world upside down and left me with what felt like no one. The rage I felt inside of me was like a brewing volcano about to erupt, and I didn't know how to hold back the explosion. I didn't want to talk to anyone about it because, one, they probably wouldn't know what to say, and two, I was so worried about people thinking that I was seeking out sympathy when I wasn't. Shannon was the only person I felt comfortable talking to about it without feeling judged. She never sugar-coated anything, but she always knew what to say to make me feel a little better.

"I just don't understand how she could leave me like that, knowing that I was going to be the one to come home and find her."

It didn't matter how angry I was, I always tried so hard to make excuses for her, to try and put myself in her shoes.

"But I know she wasn't thinking clearly about what she was doing, and in that moment, she just wanted it all to stop."

Shannon let out a huge sigh.

"I know what she did was not fair, and that's all there is to it. But I know that one day, you will find peace within yourself and be able to forgive her."

I nodded.

"But what if I become as unhappy as she was and don't want to be here anymore?" I asked. I was deeply petrified of becoming just like her.

"Ebonie, you are not your mum. You are your own person, and you have so much life ahead of you to be excited about," she reassured me. I took a deep breath in and smiled softly, knowing that she was right. I was my own person, and I was determined to make my mum proud.

Of course, the world didn't stop turning, and life went on. I continued to play, laugh and have fun. But every time I caught myself experiencing a moment of joy, I was struck with an immediate sting of guilt.

How can I be happy at a time like this? I shouldn't be laughing. I shouldn't be having fun without Mum, I'd think. I had no idea what I was supposed to feel, which emotions were allowed, and which ones weren't.

I stayed with my neighbours for the first few weeks after my mum passed. I wasn't ready to leave what I knew as home, to sleep in a new bed, or not be able to simply pop next door to play with my best friend anymore.

I opened the front door and nervously stepped back inside my house for the first time since I'd found my mum after weeks of avoiding it at all costs. I had the urge to remove my shoes, even though she wasn't there to tell me off anymore. I did it anyway, out of some sort of respect for her. The strength of her natural, earthy scent filled my nostrils as I took a deep breath in and walked slowly down the hallway, feeling the cold, hard terracotta tiles underneath my feet. When I reached the kitchen, I immediately noticed the curtains on my right had been tightly closed to cover up the view to the outdoor patio – I wasn't ready to face that just yet.

I stood quietly in the middle of the dining room, observing the space around me and becoming increasingly aware of the smallest of details: the placement of the remote control on the coffee table next to the couch, the dishes by the sink that hadn't been put away yet, the chair by the dining room table that was clearly out of place after I'd pushed it aside in my panic to get to her. I could feel my body starting to tremble and my pulse beginning to skyrocket as the memories came flooding back. I wasn't sure how much longer I could stay there.

I was then hit with the realisation that the house didn't feel like my home anymore. I felt like I'd fallen into a deep hole, in free fall. All I wanted to do was drop to the ground and beg for my mum to come back. I no longer knew where I belonged; where my home was. I felt completely lost and alone, and the one person I wanted to rescue me would now only ever be a series of memories.

"Home is not a house, a city or a place. It's where you feel most able to be yourself. And it's the people you feel most able to be yourself with."

– Mark Manson

15

Aunty Jan and Rex had been married for fourteen years before they were sprung with the unforeseeable news they now had a twelve-year-old child and her dog coming to live with them permanently. Obviously, Bella and I were a package deal. She had been a gift from my mum and was a significant part of what felt like home.

Aunty Jan and Rex lived in a very small and quaint, two-bed, one-bath cottage that was built on a beautiful four-acre block of land with a dam down the back – the perfect home for families of ducks and their offspring. They adored this house, particularly the tranquillity and peacefulness of being out in the countryside, yet only a five or ten-minute drive to reach anything you'd ever need.

Prior to me, being a parent was not a role that Aunty Jan and Rex were very familiar with. Although they tried for many years, unfortunately, they never got the opportunity to have children of their own; instead, they were blessed with a grieving, traumatised and very vulnerable almost teenager – the perfect combination.

Rex had known me since the day I was born; he had held me in his arms as a baby and watched me become more like my mum year after year. But I didn't share the same bond with Rex that I had with Aunty Jan, and I found it really difficult to connect with him on a deeper level. When Aunty Jan wasn't around to mediate the conversation, I often found myself feeling very awkward and unsure of what to say. I felt so guilty for the lack of conversation with him, but unfortunately, his passion for restoring old stationary engines was not something we had in common.

* * * * *

Their charismatic Queenslander was the first house to be built in their street over a century ago, which meant there was always some sort of renovation going on to maintain its appeal. They had been planning on adding an extension onto the house for a while before I came to live with them, and Rex was determined to complete this masterpiece himself, from start to finish.

Rex was a quiet achiever, the type of guy who never felt the need to boast about his successes in order to feel good about himself. He worked as a mechanic for most of his life and had an unending enthusiasm for anything with a motor. On his days off, if he wasn't inside the house watching his favourite motorbike racer, Casey Stoner, or looking up which shares in the stock market were rising or falling, he was outside working on one of his multiple projects – building a new bedroom being one of them.

It took twelve months of uninterrupted dedication and persistence for Rex to achieve this mammoth task, and there stood a large square-shaped room that was almost the size of the house itself. A space that was cleverly designed to match the antique feel of its surrounding walls, with a modern and revitalising twist; a room that somehow became mine.

When I took my first steps onto the timeless natural hardwood flooring, my eyes were immediately drawn to the turquoise feature wall at the back, which instantly lifted my spirits. Our voices echoed as they bounced off the off-white textured wall panels, helping to create an even brighter, more spacious atmosphere. I walked over to the French wooden double doors that opened out onto the back deck and noticed our neighbour's perfectly groomed show horse reaching its long, slender neck over the wired fence, munching on the green grass that was surely no different to what was on his side. The room joined the rest of the house via a door that led to the kitchen and lounge area, as well as a separate door to the old spare room, which later became my ensuite: a tiny bedroom but a rather large bathroom. I considered myself to be one lucky thirteen-year-old. This room became my safe haven, a space that made me feel calm and at peace with my thoughts when nowhere else did.

* * * * *

After leaving my childhood home behind and moving in permanently with Aunty Jan and Rex, I soon realised that it wasn't just my life that had been completely turned upside down. Their lives had been too.

Mum and Aunty Jan were best of friends; however, they were opposites in many ways. My mum had a typical type A personality; she was an extroverted, stubborn, ambitious perfectionist who spent most of her time being hyper-aware of all the things she had not yet done for the day, and on the contrary, Aunty Jan was like a breath of fresh air. She was far more laid back, patient and flexible in her approach to life.

Although Aunty Jan was trying her best to maintain as much consistency in my life as she could in a way that was similar to how it was with my mum, her parenting style was nothing like what I was used to. She never got angry or felt the need to raise her voice at me, but instead, she would try to express herself more calmly and gently, which only seemed to wind me up even more.

* * * * *

I was back in Shannon's office, trying to figure out a way to articulate my emotions into words. The numbness I felt deep within my soul lasted for weeks following my mum's passing – to be expected. It was like a bomb had exploded right in front of me, and I was trying my best to navigate through the debris to figure out what this new way of life looked like.

"I feel like I can't yell at Aunty Jan like my mum and I used to yell and scream at each other. It's like I have to be on my best behaviour all the time." I began to express my current struggles to Shannon as I sat with my shoulders hunched forward and my arms gently crossed in my lap.

"What happens when you do get angry with her?" Shannon asked.

"I get annoyed and say a few things, but mostly, I try to hold it all in and just go straight to my room to be alone." This had become my new way of coping.

"Sometimes I'll slam my door to try to let out some of my anger, but it never feels like enough."

The fury I felt deep inside of me made me want to scream at the top of my lungs and smash any inanimate object I could get my hands on, but instead, I would find myself sitting in my room on the hardwood floorboards while my emotions continued to boil up inside of me. Sometimes, I'd be sitting with my head resting in my hands, breathing heavily to calm myself down. Other times, I thought about just giving up completely.

It would take hours for me to feel comfortable enough to emerge from my room and talk to her again.

"Why don't you feel like you can tell her how you're really feeling at that moment?" She asked, inviting me to delve deeper into my frustrations, but I think she already knew my answer.

"I feel too guilty afterwards. I know she has just taken on this huge role of looking after me, and it's not like it was something she wanted, but she didn't really have a choice."

I couldn't help but feel like an orphan child who had just been dumped on their front doorstep without any prior warning and no instruction manual on how to raise a grieving thirteen-year-old.

"I feel like a burden," I whispered and looked down at my hands as the tears in my eyes got heavier.

"I understand why you feel that way, but Aunty Jan and Rex always had a choice. Taking responsibility for you was not forced upon them; they wanted to."

I knew deep down this was true, but I was really struggling to believe it.

"Your task is not to seek for love, but merely to seek and find all the barriers within yourself that you have built against it."

– Rumi

16

Every morning on our way to school, Aunty Jan and I would drive past the same lonely house on a hill with no neighbours nearby. There stood the sweetest-looking, stumpy-legged miniature pony who was just too cute not to notice. Day after day, we saw him tethered to a rope that was no more than ten metres long, to the same tree that he'd wrap himself around multiple times, leaving no slack to be able to move freely. His nose was constantly glued to the ground as he searched tirelessly amongst the dry, uneven, dusty surface for the strands of green grass that were almost non-existent. His owners had clearly neglected him and Aunty Jan felt incredibly sorry for him.

A few weeks went by, and the pony's barrel of a stomach was

starting to get smaller, his eyes were looking sadder, and his thick dark brown coat was becoming duller. Aunty Jan wanted to do anything she could to help, so she decided to buy a bale of hay that she stored in the boot of our car, and almost every afternoon on her way to pick me up from school, she would take a small section, and hand feed it to him.

As Aunty Jan was driving past one afternoon, she noticed the owner of the pony and her two daughters standing on their front porch. She parked the car in their driveway and made her way towards them.

"Hi there, my name is Jan," she said. There was no return greeting.

The lady appeared to be a little rough around the edges; she was holding a cigarette in one hand and a large glass of wine in the other at four o'clock in the afternoon.

"I just love your pony; he is so cute!" Jan tried again. "I just wanted to let you know that I've got plenty of grass at my place and a lot of free space, so if you ever want to bring him around, you are more than welcome. I only live up the road."

She smiled, but the lady made it clear she was not interested in Aunty Jan's offer in the slightest.

"He is fine, just where he is," her cold and unwelcoming tone spoke volumes to Aunty Jan. Unfortunately, the situation was out of her control.

A few weeks later, Aunty Jan's wish had been granted when she drove past for the thousandth time and saw a 'Pony for Sale' sign at the front of their house.

'This is my chance to rescue him and give him the love and care he deserves,' she thought.

We were sitting around the dinner table later that evening when Aunty Jan decided that it was time to test the waters and ask Rex about the possibility of buying the pony. She explained the situation to him, making it sound a little more dramatic than it was, with high hopes that it would persuade him to give her the answer she so badly wanted to hear.

"No, sweetie, we are not buying a pony."

Rex was not an animal lover to begin with, and his logical mind could not see the point in buying a pony for the sake of it. In his eyes, he was simply not our problem.

In the following weeks, she asked another two more times, and to her disappointment, he would not budge. Meanwhile, the pony remained in the same spot, gradually becoming more malnourished and looking more distressed as time passed by.

One afternoon, Rex arrived home from work and was unexpectedly welcomed home by a new friend, who looked just as confused as he was. Aunty Jan was calmly brushing his dusty, matted coat under the house when Rex walked up to the fence with a stunned look on his face.

"So, who do we have here?" he asked sarcastically, knowing exactly what she'd done.

"Meet Bluey! But don't worry, he won't be staying; I just had to rescue him from where he was," Jan said hurriedly.

Bluey let out a high-pitched neigh, nodding his head up and down in approval of what he thought was his new home.

Rex stood there, quietly observing the beautiful connection that Aunty Jan had formed with Bluey and immediately saw how much joy he brought into her world. Five minutes went by, and he turned to her.

"He is quite cute. I think we should keep him," Rex said.

Aunty Jan looked up at him in complete disbelief; her face lit up like a Christmas tree.

"Really?" She looked back down at Bluey with the biggest grin on her face and nudged her cheek against his muzzle.

"Bluey, welcome to our family!"

It was in moments like these when Aunty Jan knew Rex was truly willing to do anything to make her happy.

"Some people are going to leave, but that's not the end of your story. That's the end of their part in your story."

– Faraaz Kazi

17

Prank-calling random people in my contact list always seemed like a good idea when I was with my friends, and we felt like being a little mischievous. It was my fourteenth birthday, and Aunty Jan had allowed me to invite four of my friends over for a sleepover, which was more than I was ever permitted when I lived with my mum. It felt odd, but in a good way.

We were sitting on my bed, looking through the contact lists on our phones, trying to decide who to call next.

"Let's prank call my dad!" I eagerly suggested.

Earlier that day, I had received a text message from him wishing me a happy birthday. We were still in contact, but it was limited to the occasional message for birthdays and Christmas. He didn't seem to want anything more. We used my phone to make the call, which, of course, had my number blocked, and we nervously waited for my dad to pick up.

"Hello?" he answered.

"Hi, um, I've lost my puppy, and I was just wondering if you've seen it?"

My friend spoke in a high-pitched, childish voice and decided to use a story that we thought seemed somewhat believable while the rest of us sat there trying to hold our giggles in.

"Yeah, we found it. And then we ate it," my dad answered abruptly before proceeding to laugh with his girlfriend, who sounded like she was sitting beside him.

My smiling lips suddenly dropped, and I looked up at my friend in shock at his choice of words, unsure of what she was going to say next. She tried to go along with the story for a little longer, but it just seemed to make things worse.

"Ebonie. Is that you?" He asked sternly, and it was obvious that he was no longer joking around.

I ripped the phone out of my friend's hand and immediately ended the call. Shit.

"How did he know it was me? And why did he sound so angry? It was just a joke."

"They sounded drunk," my friend replied.

A few moments later, my phone buzzed, and I looked down to see a text from him. I reluctantly picked up my phone and opened the message.

'Ebonie, I know that was you and your friends on the phone. Don't ever fucking contact me again. I never want to fucking speak to you or see you again.'

My eyes widened, and my heart felt like it had lurched into the base of my throat.

My phone buzzed again.

'You're a dropkick entity just like your fucked up mother.'

My blood began to boil as I read his harsh words. I wanted to yell and scream and cry all at the same time. It was one thing to call me names and tell me to fuck off but to disrespect my mother like that and then compare me to her was low, really low.

What was meant to be an enjoyable night celebrating my birthday quickly turned into me feeling like an absolute idiot in front of my friends, as well as ruining any kind of relationship I had left with my dad. My response was just as childish, and he probably read it and laughed, but I was done with him. He had really hurt me this time, and I despised him for that.

"People do not decide their futures,
they decide their habits and their
habits decide their futures."

– F. M. Alexander

18

I was fifteen years old when I stood on the scales one morning and realised that I was the heaviest I'd ever been. I felt disgusting. I hated the way I looked in the mirror, how I looked in photos, and the extra padding I held around my thighs and my belly.

It then became a morning ritual for me to step on the scales, instantly feel shit about myself and then stand in front of the mirror and continue picking apart all the things I disliked about my body.

My stomach isn't flat enough, I'd think. My muscles aren't toned enough. My thighs are touching. At some point, I decided that having a 'thigh gap' was the thing that determined whether my legs were thin enough. I would sit on my bed at night with my knees bent and touching to see if I had a gap between my legs yet.

It was at this time that my dancing days came to an end, and I decided that I wanted to try something different, something that was a little more physically demanding, to help me lose some of my pudginess.

I joined a local under-sixteen girls' Australian Football League team around the time when women's AFL was starting to become more popular, a couple of years before the first official women's league was announced in 2017. I had grown up watching this sport with my mum and had always wanted to give it a try – this was the perfect opportunity.

Although I was extremely nervous to start, my love for playing the sport grew rapidly and to my surprise, my football skills actually weren't too shabby. I was rewarded the best and fairest trophy at the end of my first season and qualified for two different Queensland state teams throughout the years I played.

Meanwhile, my unspoken goal of losing weight began to consume my every thought. Exercise became a means of burning more calories so that I could allow myself to eat more, and my ability to enjoy food for what it was took a very steep downward spiral.

For months I continued to stare at the number on the scales in disbelief.

How can the number still be going up when I'm exercising so hard and practically starving myself? I wondered.

I began to feel as though I had completely lost control over my body, and I didn't know how to get it back. I started to eliminate all the foods that I thought were causing me to gain weight – carbs and fats being a huge portion of that.

I would spend way too much time in the supermarket looking at the nutrition labels on everything I bought. If the calories were too high, the item would immediately go back on the shelf without a second thought. I didn't care if the alternative I chose didn't taste as good; I just wanted the lowest calorie option: low-fat yogurt, unsweetened almond milk, canned tuna in spring water, low-carb bread, high protein pasta, sugar-free maple syrup… the list went on.

The kitchen scales and the My Fitness Pal app became my new best friends, which I used religiously to track everything. I even started to weigh my spinach leaves – a rough estimate wasn't good enough.

I took charge of packing my lunches for school so that I knew exactly what I was eating and how much. I tried to weigh my food as discretely as possible so that Aunty Jan wouldn't notice. But she always did. I packed an apple and a muesli bar for morning tea, which I didn't eat until I had removed every single chocolate chip from the top. My lunch was usually some form of chicken salad or leftovers from the night before. When I got home from school, starving, I would indulge in a handful of carrot sticks and then force myself to wait until dinner to eat again.

It took months for my body to get the memo and finally start to shed some kilos, but the relief I felt was rejuvenating.

My body isn't broken!

I told myself that when I reached the weight I had in mind, I would be happy; I would be proud of the girl I saw in the mirror.

The day I stepped onto the scales and saw the magic number that I had been working so hard to achieve for so long was the day that I finally felt worthy again. It was a feeling of satisfaction that very quickly became addictive.

I continued to over-exercise, eat the same few calories I was used to and weighed myself day after day. The number kept creeping lower and lower, and although I was no longer 'intentionally' losing weight, deep down, I was proud of it.

After two years of playing footy, I decided to move on and join a gym instead so that I could direct my focus on my last two years of high school.

I had lost a total of thirteen kilos, and at this point, I was borderline anorexic.

The insistent fear of putting on weight again meant that my appearance took priority over anything else, and my physical health took a back seat. I became significantly iron and B12 deficient, my hormones were completely out of whack, and my energy levels were at an all-time low. My menstrual cycle disappeared, and I was later diagnosed with hypothalamic amenorrhea, a condition that develops as a result of poor nutrition, stress or too much exercise – I was currently ticking all of those boxes. My body was essentially telling me that I was not healthy enough to carry a baby, so it stopped producing the hormones required to trigger the onset of a period. I knew that none of this was healthy and it could have a serious impact on my long-term health, but I chose to focus more on how I looked. That was my only priority, everything else was a future me problem.

Social events started to make me anxious. I couldn't go out for a meal with my friends without first knowing where we were going, then looking up the menu online, deciding exactly what I was going to order, and adapting the rest of my daily intake around that specific meal to make sure I was within my calorie target.

If I ordered a meal, I was that person who would have at least one request: salad dressing on the side, no butter on the toast, and no cheese on the pizza. My friends who didn't understand would look at me like I was from another planet for removing the tastiest parts of the dish. I was embarrassed but I couldn't help it.

If the meal came out and didn't meet my expectations, or the online menu was different to the menu I had in front of me, my entire mood would change. I would feel myself draw inwards, like a turtle retracting itself back into its shell. I hated being so difficult; I so badly wanted to be like everyone else, to be able to order a meal without overanalysing every single ingredient.

My anxiety around food, exercise and my body image continued to intensify, spiralling into something I felt like I'd lost control over, and I didn't know where it was all coming from.

"The capacity to learn is a gift; the ability to learn is a skill; the willingness to learn is a choice."

– Brian Herbert

19

When it came to learning how to drive, choosing a reliable car, or knowing how to check the car's engine oil, I was very grateful to have Rex. The day I turned sixteen, I took my learner's driving test, and thankfully, after completing the online practice quiz hundreds of times, I passed with flying colours.

I had saved enough money to buy myself a second-hand navy blue, four-door Suzuki Swift. Her given name was Swifty and she was Rex approved. Learning to drive a manual was absolutely not my idea of fun. It took me months to be able to successfully drive one hundred metres up the road and change gears without bunny-hopping the entire way and then coming to a rather abrupt halt. I'd get so fed up that I'd get out of the car, slam the door and yell, 'fuck this!' to which Aunty Jan's response would be to quickly get out of the passenger seat and back in front of the steering wheel. Aunty Jan was the one who got to deal with me losing my temper. For some reason, I was far more mellow and calm while practising with Rex, probably because I felt slightly less comfortable around him and didn't want to embarrass myself. But he was always so calm, and he had an incredible amount of patience; it made me feel like I couldn't ever give up. He helped me with the most complex of driving skills that made me the most nervous: how to reverse in a straight line, do a parallel park, and complete a three-point turn in three manoeuvres, not ten. Every time I made a mistake, he'd say, 'That's okay, let's try again,' without blinking an eyelid.

Twelve months and one hundred hours of supervised driving later, on my seventeenth birthday, I was finally able to take my provisional driving test. I didn't want to wait a day longer to gain my independence, and I'm sure Aunty Jan and Rex were just as excited to have their freedom back after five years of being my personal Uber driver seven days a week.

Thirty minutes into the test, I had completed a hill start, a three-point turn and a U-turn, and then my examiner asked me to execute a reverse in a straight line. Shit, I hate this one.

"It's okay, take your time." My examiner had somehow heard my thoughts and could tell how nervous I was. I took a deep breath in, turned my head to look over my left shoulder and tried to recall Rex's cues in my head, as I reversed the car as perfectly as I could until my examiner ordered me to stop.

When we arrived back at the parking lot, I turned off the car engine, let out a sigh of relief, and waited patiently for him to finish signing off the paperwork to find out my result. He had maintained a straight face the entire time and was clearly determined not to give anything away. My armpits were sweating, and my heart was beating one hundred miles an hour; the suspense was killing me.

Finally, he put his pen down and looked over at me with very little expression on his face.

"I almost had to fail you at the end there, but you stopped inside the line just in time. Congratulations, Ebonie, you have passed," he grinned.

My smile could not have been any bigger. My freedom was finally here.

"Darkness cannot drive out darkness;
only light can do that."

– Martin Luther King Jr.

20

It felt invigorating to finally be able to drive myself to school on the first day of my last year of high school and park up next to the rest of the cohort who already had their licence. I was feeling refreshed and motivated for the year ahead after a well-deserved eight-week break, but also very keen to graduate and move on to bigger and better things, like university.

I had always described myself as a floater at school; I was never one of the super popular girls, but I got along with almost everyone, and I liked it that way. My school was small, with about one hundred and twenty students in each grade, separated into four classrooms. My grade was quite a close group; we all knew each other well, and nothing went unnoticed, especially if there was a new kid in town.

My eyes were immediately drawn to his beautifully bronzed skin and short blonde hair that was just long enough for the breeze to catch it as he walked through the school corridor, accompanied by one of the teachers who was showing him to his locker. He wore his brand new, freshly ironed white blouse and navy blue shorts, with his perfectly knotted tie and long navy socks pulled up to exactly where they were supposed to be. He was about the same height as me, lean and well-built, with broad shoulders and rather defined biceps that bulged through the sleeves of his shirt. He was clearly into sport of some sort and was very nice on the eyes, but I knew that's all he'd ever be. He would never go for a girl like me.

It was the night of our year twelve formal, and I was being accompanied by one of my best mates who had asked me to be his formal partner towards the end of the previous year. I was wearing an elegant dark purple sequinned gown that gently hugged the sides of my body and complemented my dark brunette hair which was tied back into a messy low bun. My makeup had been beautifully done, with a gentle contour, smoky black eyes, and finished with bright red lipstick. I felt beautiful.

I was standing at the front of the line with my girlfriends, waiting to get our professional photos taken in front of the bronze material backdrop, jealously watching as Sam had his photo taken with about five different girls, wishing that one of them was with me. My eyes locked with his as he stepped to the side of the backdrop, and my heart fluttered at the unexpected eye contact. I smiled awkwardly at him as he made his way towards me.

"Did you want to get a photo?" he asked. A smile tugged at the corners of my mouth and the butterflies began to actively dance around in my stomach.

"Yeah, sure," I replied as cool, calm and collected as I could; little did he know that was all I wanted.

Sam was in my math class and sat a few seats down from me. He could tell that I was the academic type from the million and one questions I would ask our teacher every lesson, but I'm pretty sure he knew that I was no genius. Math was not my best subject, but it very quickly became one of my favourites.

"Eb, can you please help me with this question?" he asked, pointing down at his textbook with a smile I could have stared at all day.

Is this guy seriously asking me for help with trigonometry? I thought.

I eagerly jumped up out of my seat and went over to his desk, hoping that I'd be able to help but also wanting to take advantage of any excuse to be next to him.

Little did I know every time he asked for my help was the perfect excuse for him to get my attention, and it worked.

It didn't come as a surprise to me when Sam figured out that I liked him without me having to say the words. I was always so awkward when it came to flirting, but I was also terrible at hiding it when I liked someone. I would send him a message to ask about some piece of homework, but always with an ulterior motive, hopeful that it would lead to a more interesting conversation.

I was lying in bed on a school night, just about to fall asleep, when I heard my phone begin to vibrate on my bedside table. I propped myself up onto my elbow and looked over, suddenly feeling very confused when I saw it was Sam who was calling me.

Is this a mistake? I wondered.

Part of me didn't want to answer because I didn't know what to say, but the temptation of hearing his voice took over. Not wanting to seem too desperate, I let it ring for a few more seconds before pressing the green button.

An hour went by, and he somehow managed to get me to admit

that I did, in fact, have a thing for him. The butterflies were back, and I could feel the heat rushing to my cheeks when he eventually admitted that he liked me, too. I wasn't sure if I'd heard him right, but I honestly couldn't have been happier.

* * * * *

A couple of months had gone by, and Sam had driven us up the mountains to a special lookout that he wanted to show me. The air was fresh, and the tranquil ambience filled the silence as he stood behind me with his arms wrapped around my waist, looking out at the beautiful panoramic view.

He rested his chin gently on my shoulder, and I could hear the softness of his breath as he slowly breathed in and out. I wanted this moment to last forever.

After a few moments, he took a deep breath in as if he was preparing himself for something.

"Eb, will you be my girlfriend?" he whispered in my ear, and I could feel the rate of his breath begin to speed up as he waited in anticipation for my response. I closed my eyes and felt myself melt into his arms before I turned around to face him and look directly into his moonlit eyes.

"Yes," I whispered before wrapping my arms around his shoulders, holding him as tight as I could. I was the happiest I'd been in a long time.

"Sometimes you won't find the closure you are looking for. Sometimes closure will find you simply in the way of moving forward, without any explanation, without all the answers, and it is still just as beautiful."

– Charlotte Freeman

21

Graduation was fast approaching, and it had been almost four years since I had last spoken to my dad when he told me never to contact him again. Although I knew the chances were slim, I thought maybe he would want to be there for this fairly significant event in my life. Perhaps he was waiting for me to be the first one to reach out after the way things ended.

I knew that he was never going respond to a text or a phone call, that the only way I would have any chance of rekindling our relationship was to find out his address and go directly to his house so that I could see him face to face. I wasn't sure if this was a good or bad idea, but at this point, I knew I had nothing to lose, and I was willing to try anything to get his attention. Every inch of me hoped that deep down, he still loved me, that he would want me back in his life if he knew that I wanted to be in his. It was worth a try.

When I told Aunty Jan about my plan, I was relieved to hear that she was on board with the idea and was willing to help in any way she could. I knew that he was living with Julie, most likely in the same house I'd visited all those years ago, but I had no idea how to get there.

I got in contact with my dad's sister, an aunt who I was very close to as a young child. I'd been to visit her, as well as my nana and grandad, in New Zealand on numerous occasions but our relationship had also become fairly distanced over the years.

I felt a glimmer of hope sweep through me when I read her response to my message, telling me that she would have a look for his home address in her address book, but that quickly disappeared when I read the second part of her message that said she didn't give out other people's personal information without their permission. This was completely fair, and I respected her intentions, but he was my dad, and I'd hoped that she would have made an exception to this personal policy of hers. Unfortunately, she didn't.

He was never going to allow her to give me his address, but I also didn't want him to know anything about it. I planned to spontaneously turn up at his front door. 'Surprise! Remember me?'

Later that evening, I was sitting at the dinner table with Aunty Jan and Rex, brainstorming other ways that I could potentially find his address when I received a text message... from my dad. My stomach dropped to the floor, and I suddenly lost my appetite.

'Ebonie, I don't care if you speak to my family but don't you dare use them to get into contact with me. Don't bother finding out where I live. You are not welcome here.'

I didn't even know how to feel. Although I knew it wasn't her fault, I was angry that my aunty had said something to my dad and basically turned my plan upside down; I was hurt because even after four years of zero contact, he was still holding onto so much anger towards me. And I was sad because I had just destroyed any chance of having my father back in my life, let alone at my graduation. He didn't even know why I was trying to contact him, nor did he want to.

He still wanted nothing to do with me, and I guess it was the closure I was searching for.

* * * * *

Twelve-year-old me would never have expected to graduate from high school with a reputation of receiving an academic award at the end of each year, and I was incredibly proud to be finishing my schooling years, far exceeding all expectations I had for myself.

By the end of my last ever school Celebration Evening, a formal event that is held at the end of every year for students to celebrate their academic, non-academic and sporting achievements, I had walked away with an academic distinction award, the subject award for biology, and the principals award – an award that recognises a student who strives for excellence in all aspects of their schooling, one who is devoted to their studies, is hardworking, reliable and an honourable role model to other students. Out of the entire grade of students, I could not believe that I had been acknowledged as this person, leaving me with the cheesiest grin that was impossible to wipe off my face.

These achievements never came easy to me. I was never one of those naturally intelligent kids who could read something once and never have to look at it again. I had to put a lot of hours into my study: writing essays, working with a math tutor, staying back after class to go over what I didn't understand, and submitting additional drafts just so that I could have a better chance at improving my final grade. I was relieved to know that all my efforts, the last five years of hard work and dedication, had paid off. On some level, I always knew my mum was there with me every step of the way. She gave me the push I needed and never let me fail. I knew that even though she was not physically there, her spiritual presence always was. It's a feeling that I'll never be able to describe. If you know, you know.

* * * * *

I enrolled into my chosen university course straight after I graduated from high school, giving myself no time to mess about. I was accepted into a Bachelor of Science at the University of Queensland, and out of the twenty-five different majors I could have chosen from, I randomly decided that I wanted to major in genetics – maybe I would be that person who discovers something life-changing, I thought.

Prior to making this big life decision, I had been told on multiple occasions that it didn't matter if I changed my mind or switched courses, that it was okay not to know exactly what career path I wanted to pursue. But in my mind, time was precious, and I didn't want to waste it. I had always enjoyed learning about the human body. Biology and chemistry were my favourite subjects, and I knew it was something I was relatively good at, so I was pretty set on my decision.

In spite of my initial enthusiasm, it didn't take me long after enrolling into university to realise it wasn't quite the right path. Spending my days in a research laboratory in a white lab coat and safety goggles, staring patiently into a microscope lens, and then waiting months or even years to make a new discovery, was not my idea of fun.

To my disappointment, I ended up changing my mind three times during my first year. From wanting to be a psychologist to a dietician to a sports scientist, I was really struggling to narrow it down to a single profession that I knew would encompass all of my passions into one. I needed some guidance. I booked an appointment with an academic advisor in my faculty, who introduced me to a degree that I didn't even know existed: a career that would allow me to help a wide range of people in more ways than one, a degree that gave me the options I was searching for; a Bachelor of Clinical Exercise Physiology.

*"Life isn't about the things that happen to you,
it's about what you do with them when they do."*

– Ryan Holiday

22

It was the beginning of 2015 and Rex had started to notice that walking up the set of stairs that led to our front door was getting slightly more difficult.

"My legs feel like they are getting weaker as the days go by. The joys of getting old," he joked one night at the dinner table. Although he was always fairly active, specific exercise was not part of his daily routine. So, in hopes of preventing the somewhat normal muscle degeneration that comes with age, or at least slowing this process down, he bought a stationary exercise bike that lived inside our house by the front door. Every day, without fail, he would complete twenty minutes of continuous cycling at a fairly high resistance. Sometimes, he'd spice things up a bit and do some high-intensity interval training to feel a little extra burn in his legs. He was determined to regain his strength again.

After three months of perseverance, there was no sign of improvement. In fact, the strength in his legs seemed to be getting worse – getting up out of a chair was getting harder, and walking up the stairs was getting slower. Something wasn't quite right, and we were all getting a little concerned.

Rex took himself off to see our family doctor, who, after viewing his blood test results, discovered that he was significantly deficient in vitamin B12, which can subsequently affect the nervous system and cause muscle weakness – he was administered a B12 infusion, and fortunately, things seemed to stabilise.

He continued with his exercise bike regime, aimed for at least ten thousand steps a day, completely gave up drinking alcohol and ate incredibly well.

Two years later, after many visits to his doctor, a number of blood tests, and regular B12 infusions, Rex continued to notice a slow but progressive decline in his strength. He was frustrated and confused. Rex's doctor requested he have a muscle biopsy to further investigate, in the hopes it would give us more clarity about what was going on.

In 2017, Rex was finally diagnosed with inclusion body myositis (IBM), a very rare condition that causes the body's immune system to turn against itself, damaging its own muscle tissue in an autoimmune process. The cause of IBM remains unclear, and unfortunately, there is no cure. This news was devastating. Rex's health had always been one of his top priorities. It was difficult to fathom that he, of all people, had ended up with this awful diagnosis. Nonetheless, he did not give up. Rex was determined to fight it. He spent hours researching his condition, trying to find new and alternative ways to reverse or slow down its progression. He was willing to try anything, but most importantly, he knew that he had to change his mindset. He became the most positive man I knew.

Unfortunately, Rex's condition continued to decline; his legs were getting weaker, and the strength in his arms and hands was also starting to deteriorate. Day after day, he started to become more aware of the simple things in life that people so often take for granted. The days of effortlessly walking up the flight of fifteen stairs in under twenty seconds were gone. It now took upwards of a minute while he gripped tightly onto the handrails and put a significant amount of his body weight through his arms to help him up each step. Opening a jar, standing up from the toilet, getting out of bed, and stepping over the ledge to get into the shower are simple everyday tasks that most people Rex's age could still do without a second thought. The homestead was becoming more and more challenging for Rex to live comfortably. It took time for Rex to come to terms with the reality of his condition, accepting that he would eventually not be able to walk up the stairs at all, but moving away from their forever home was never a consideration in his mind. So, something else needed to be done.

This was when the biggest project of them all began, and unfortunately, it was not one that Rex was able to physically assist with. They decided to build a second house on the same property: a modern, Hamptons-style, three-bedroom, three-bathroom home that would be completely accessible for Rex. By the time this house was ready to move into, twelve months later, Rex was finally ready to say goodbye to the home he loved so dearly.

"You can't go back and change the beginning, but you can start where you are and change the ending."

– C.S Lewis

23

While Rex was having his battles, I was having mine. It had been one year since I'd graduated from high school, and my disordered eating patterns were at their peak. It was consuming every part of me. My body was beginning to look extremely weak; my face was drawn, my ribs were more prominent, and I now had a thigh gap almost the size of a tennis ball. I was aware of my habits, and I knew they were unhealthy, but I didn't know how to switch them off. I needed help.

I took myself to see Shannon again, desperately hoping that she would be able to help me understand how I had gotten to this dark and scary place.

I sat down in the same black leather armchair that she had on my last visit three years ago and started from where we had left off. My palms were sweating as I fiddled with my fingers and looked down at the rug beneath my feet. I could feel the anxiety beaming out of my chest.

"My whole life has revolved around numbers: how much I weigh, how many calories I eat, how many grams of protein I'm getting, how much my chicken weighs, the circumference measure of my stomach and thighs. I can't take it anymore. I just want it all to stop!" I rubbed my hands over my eyes in frustration before looking up at Shannon with eyes of desperation, wanting her to just wave a magic wand and take it all away.

"What would happen if you were to eat a Mars bar or if you were to put on a couple of kilos?" Shannon's brows furrowed as she asked me this very simple question.

I sat in silence for a few moments, staring out the window to the left of her chair.

"Probably nothing," I finally admitted. "I don't know why I do this to myself, and every time I feel like I've got a handle on it, it likes to remind me that I really haven't. I hate it." I could feel myself wanting to scream and cry all at the same time.

"I feel like this whole thing has become a significant part of my identity, and I almost don't know who I am without it," I confessed.

"Ebonie, it's important to realise that this eating disorder hasn't come out of nowhere; it is simply how your trauma has manifested itself on a surface level, and to be able to truly make a difference, we need to try to understand the root cause of it."

After a few moments of talking, I remembered how safe I used to feel in this small room, the only place where I felt safe enough to express my deepest and darkest thoughts.

With Shannon's guidance, I began to unzip the large suitcase of emotions that I had stored away for so many years, slowly revealing the unwanted feelings that I'd buried so deep beneath the surface that I'd completely forgotten about them. I was almost disappointed that they were still there, waiting to be found.

We continued to dig so deep that I eventually reached the bottom of the bag, and all of a sudden, my mind and body felt completely at ease. I had finally found the missing piece to the puzzle.

"I don't feel good enough, not even for myself," I blurted out, and my eyes began to weep.

"How can I be worthy of anyone if the two most important people in my life chose to leave me?" The tears now rolled down my cheeks, and it was at that moment that I came to realise the why behind this debilitating mental disorder. It hadn't just developed for no reason; it was simply a product of my past.

My dad loved me once but no longer wanted me in his life. My mum had decided to give up and leave her entire life behind. In a way that felt like she had given up on me, too. I had no control over what happened to me, over who decided to stay in my life or who didn't. I was left feeling unloved and unwanted by the people who were meant to love me unconditionally, no matter what obstacles they came across.

"Ebonie, no one will ever be able to explain or make up for what your parents have done, but I want you to realise that it never had anything to do with you. You were just caught up in a very dysfunctional family." Shannon tried to reassure me.

I knew this deep down. Very deep down. But my way of coping with my disheartening subconscious beliefs was to cling onto the only thing I knew I could control, the only aspect of my life that no one could take away from me – my ability to micromanage everything I put into my mouth.

I came to realise that I didn't necessarily have a fear of putting on the weight itself but instead, I was deeply afraid of feeling like I had failed in the one area of my life that I felt I did have control over. I knew there was no one else in this world that held the same expectations that I held for myself. I needed to set myself free from this need to be so perfect in every aspect of my life, because it was this fear of failure that was beginning to eat me up inside. It just so happened that I no longer had control over it; the disorder had taken control over me.

* * * * *

"What was I like when I first came to see you?"

Shannon lifted her chin slightly and looked towards the ceiling as she tried to retrieve the memories of my first few visits six years ago.

"Well, in the first few months, you were so scared, very unsettled and didn't say much. Your whole world had just turned upside down and would never be the same again. It took a long time for you to feel more at ease and come out of your shell. We actually spent a lot of time talking about your dad and working through your emotions around him until you were ready to talk about your mum."

"I really struggle to remember a lot of the details throughout the first year or two after my mum died; I don't know why." I looked curiously at Shannon, hoping she would enlighten me on why this might be.

"That's very normal," she replied. "You were so young, and the impact of grief on someone's memory is actually quite significant. After losing a loved one, your mind is often so consumed by your memories of that person and the emotions you feel towards that tragic event that it makes it very challenging for your brain to be able to take in new information and create new memories unrelated to said grief," she explained. Suddenly, the missing pieces started to make a lot more sense.

*"The only way barriers exist is in our heads.
We create them, we feed them, and we choose
to keep them alive."*

– Katie Piper

24

After we graduated from high school, Sam and I took off to Hamilton Island, one of the most popular Whitsunday Islands located in North Queensland, next to the Great Barrier Reef, to celebrate our short-lived freedom before committing to another four years of study at university. We then made it our goal to do an overseas trip at the end of each year during our long-winded three-month uni holiday.

Our first big adventure together was a three-week holiday around different parts of Europe. We were set to arrive in London before doing a round trip through Paris, Amsterdam, Munich, Vienna, and Rome, with enough time in each place to tick off the major tourist sites. I was keen to leave the scorching summer heat behind for a few weeks but slightly worried about landing in a country that was going to be the complete opposite… freezing. I had the only winter coat I owned packed in my carry-on bag, and I hoped that I had everything else I needed to stay warm jammed in my suitcase.

The part of this trip that I was most nervous about was the food. At this point, my eating disorder had practically stolen my identity; I was tracking absolutely everything on the My Fitness Pal app, scanning bar codes and logging my salad ingredients. I was almost completely against drinking alcohol because of the 'empty calorie content', and I was extremely on edge about having no home-cooked meals and going three weeks without a gym.

But I really didn't want this to interfere with our holiday. I wanted to relax, enjoy trying all the new and traditional foods, and allow myself to have a drink every now and then simply because I felt like it. That was the plan.

* * * * *

Our days were jam-packed with all the sightseeing you could have imagined, strolling through the incredibly old but stunning cathedrals and museums, exploring the quaint and lively streets of each city, and racking up over twenty-thousand steps each day while burning enough calories just to try and stay warm.

The holiday was full of laughs, adventure, and new experiences, everything I had imagined it to be and more, until it came time to find somewhere to eat, and my anxiety began to unravel. It was like I'd hit a brick wall that I didn't know how to get around as I tried to fight against the destructive thoughts that were consuming my mind.

Don't eat too much or you'll get fat, I thought.

Save the calories so you can eat more later. Make sure you stay under your calorie budget.

I was so fixated on consuming as few calories as possible, trying to track everything I ate as best I could, but only when Sam wasn't looking. I'd wake up in the middle of the night, and my stomach would be screaming for food because I hadn't eaten enough the day before. I made myself so constipated that I ended up having to take laxatives more than once because my system was so out of whack. And the worst part was I was doing all of this to myself, and I was struggling to get through it.

* * * * *

We had arrived at our small but cozy Airbnb, located just outside of the hustle and bustle of Rome, and I was beginning to feel a little homesick; I was just about ready to fly home and return to my normal routine.

It was just after six o'clock in the evening, practically the middle of the afternoon for the Italians, but I was starving and wanted to eat dinner at that very moment.

Sam and I sat on the bed, googling nearby restaurants, trying to find one that opened before seven-thirty, a task that was far more challenging than I expected.

I was starting to feel agitated at the thought of having to wait another hour and a half before being able to sit down for a nice meal.

Of course, there was always the option of getting a pizza, a crappy takeaway or even just a light snack to keep me going, but no. I wanted to wait for something healthy, a specific menu that I could choose from. I chose to be difficult.

"Eb, what's wrong?" Sam looked over his shoulder to see that I'd given up looking and was now lying on the bed with my arms crossed and the corners of my mouth drooping to the floor.

"Nothing," I snapped. He let out a heavy sigh as he turned his head back to his phone and continued scrolling through the list of restaurants. I could tell that my attitude was beginning to get on his nerves, and although every part of me wanted to snap out of this shitty mood I'd gotten myself into, something wasn't letting me.

"I think I've got an idea. Let's go." He stood up from the bed and held out his hand to help me up.

"Where are we going?" I questioned him, hoping that he'd found a solution.

"You'll see," he smirked.

We walked for about ten minutes before stopping outside a rather fancy-looking restaurant with stairs that led up to a rooftop view.

"It opens at seven, but I think the bar is open, so we can sit and have a drink in the meantime. It was the best I could find."

Sam looked at me, desperately hoping that this would be enough to put a smile back on my face. I immediately felt a rush of guilt flow through my body for the way I had been acting.

"Thank you," I said as I reached out my hand to hold his.

"I'm so sorry." I hated the way my anxiety affected my mood and turned me into someone I really didn't want to be, but I was so grateful to have Sam by my side, willing to do anything to make me happy.

* * * * *

When I stood on the scales the morning after we arrived home, I was shocked to see that I had dropped three kilos over the three weeks we were away. I was now sitting at the lightest I'd ever been, and I was secretly happy about it.

"When you compete with people who aren't competing with you, you're simply competing with your ego. It's much healthier to focus on yourself and set personal goals to achieve – without obsessing over the idea of perfection."

– Vex King

25

While studying full-time at uni, I also decided to do my Certificate IV in Fitness, with the idea in mind of working in the health and fitness industry as a personal trainer while finishing my degree. Soon after completing my certificate, I was offered a job as a personal trainer at a brand-new gym that had just opened up not far from where I lived, within the same franchise as the gym I was already training at. I was stoked to have been given this opportunity, to be able to gain hands-on practical experience within the fitness industry that could later be used in my career as an exercise physiologist.

The process of learning how to run my own business, thinking of a unique brand name, setting up a reliable payment system, and then selling myself to clients was a very overwhelming experience at first. I was very much out of my depth, but I persisted, and with the help of my new manager, I eventually got my business up and running.

A few months into the job, I was told that my manager was leaving, and we had a new lady starting in a few weeks. Change was not something I handled well, especially when I had only just begun to settle into this new job, so I was a little apprehensive about having someone completely new take over.

* * * * *

It was eight o'clock on a Monday morning, and I was sitting at the small round table just outside the office, waiting for my next client to arrive.

The front door swung open, and I looked up from my phone to see our new manager briskly walking towards me. I got up from my chair and smiled at her.

"Good morning, I'm Ebonie," I said as I held out my hand to meet hers.

"Hello, I'm Jenny! Nice to meet you," she replied enthusiastically.

My eyes were immediately drawn to her perfectly straightened, platinum blonde hair that sat just past her shoulders before noticing her incredibly muscular figure – I had to pull my eyes away and stop myself from staring. I instantly wanted to know more about her: how she trained, what she ate, how exactly she looked the way she did.

It didn't take long for me to discover that Jenny was just as fanatic about food and exercise as I was. She had competed in multiple body-building competitions over the years, and although she wasn't currently in the preparation stages for another one, she had this impressive ability to be able to maintain a physique that was so lean and well-developed that she could've easily stepped on stage at any moment.

The more I got to know her, the more I realised I was literally a younger version of her. We were two anxious hotheads who were obsessed with the gym and over-analysed our every word, but we understood each other perfectly, and this, to me, was refreshing. Jenny and I became more than just work colleagues; our instant connection grew into a very special, long-lasting friendship that I knew I'd forever be grateful for.

* * * * *

I thoroughly enjoyed working as a personal trainer, particularly being able to have control over my hours and my rates and learn the ins and outs of how to run my own business. But it got to a stage where working split shifts every day, having clients cancel last minute, not showing up at all or needing to reschedule started to outweigh the benefits of working for myself. Building my client base and earning a consistent, reliable income while also trying to study full-time was beginning to become very difficult to manage. After eighteen months of persevering, I decided that being self-employed just wasn't the right move for me at this point in my life, and it was time for me to move on to something a little less stress-provoking: to work for someone else instead.

"It's impossible to have a successful relationship with someone else if you don't have a successful relationship with yourself."

– Danny Morel

26

I was catching up with Jenny for breakfast after our gym session together. We went to the local outlet centre down the road and chose a restaurant that we had ordered coffee from before. I decided to try something a little different on the menu, rather than my usual poached eggs and avocado on sourdough – something that was easily trackable.

When the waitress put the plate down in front of me, my eyes were immediately drawn to the oil that was dripping off the crispy kale and onto the vegetable quiche below it. Within seconds, my anxiety had made a sudden appearance:

You can't eat this; all that oil is going to undo all your hard work from this morning and make you fat.

The more rational part of my brain was trying its best to fight back.

Ebonie, it's just one meal; it's not going to make a difference. The healthy fats are good for you.

I reluctantly grabbed my knife and fork and shifted the kale to the side. I was trying to maintain my conversation with Jenny while fighting the internal battle I was having in my head at the same time. All I wanted to do was throw the meal in the bin and start again.

It's a waste of money if you don't eat it, don't be silly, I told myself.

I forced myself to eat most of it, picking my way around the oily parts while attempting to hide my anxiety. But it didn't work; Jenny could see straight through it and knew that my mood had completely changed. I honestly couldn't wait to get out of there so I could be by myself and crumble in a heap.

When I got into my car to drive home, I immediately called Sam, hoping that he would be able to rescue me from myself. He could tell how worked up I had gotten as I cried to him on the phone, and he tried his best to settle me down.

As I slid open the front door, I heard him walking out of his office. He looked at me with a comforting smile on his face and directed me to sit down with him on the couch. He wrapped his arms around my waist and pulled me in towards him.

"Eb, it was just one meal. Nothing is going to change. I promise you."

I stared into the distance and remained silent, too embarrassed to say any of what I was thinking out loud. My heart was beating rapidly, my breathing was short and sharp, and my mind had unleashed. The anxious thoughts continued to spiral.

The calories in that meal were probably so high I don't even know how to track it. I wish I just stuck to my usual order. Now, I won't be able to eat much for the rest of the day. What if I get hungry and I want to eat? I'll just have to eat a salad for dinner, no carbs and no fats.

I'll have a carrot as a snack if I get hungry.

I finally interjected my thoughts and replied to Sam.

"It was just so oily and not what I was expecting at all. I know I'm being so silly, but I can't get rid of this feeling. I wish I weren't like this," I managed. I hated what my anxiety did to me, the panic it caused me to feel over something I knew was so insignificant.

"Did you enjoy it?" Sam asked me curiously.

"Yes… It was nice," I admitted, but I didn't care about the taste. I was far more concerned about the calories.

"Sometimes it's about the experience of eating the food Eb, not just the nutritional content of it."

He knew exactly where my mind was going, and he was right. I had gotten myself so worked up about the meal itself that I hadn't even enjoyed the time with my friend.

*"Starting again doesn't mean you failed the first time.
Sometimes it means you finally worked out that
maybe things weren't quite right the way they were,
that maybe they should be better."*

– Charlotte Freeman

27

It became a regular occurrence for Jenny and I to meet at the gym on a Saturday morning to train together and catch up on the week that had been and gone.

"I really want to find a sport that gives me more of a purpose for my training, to have a goal to work towards," I began to explain to Jenny as we continued our brisk walk on the treadmills next to each other.

"I obviously love the gym, but I feel like I'm not getting anywhere with it. It's just a monotonous routine that I put myself through week after week," I continued.

"Why don't you try bikini modelling?" she suggested. "It's not as intense as the figure modelling I've done, but it's still a huge commitment and requires a lot of hard work and dedication to your training. You could easily do it."

Bodybuilding had been a huge part of Jenny's life for a long time now, and it was something she was extremely passionate about.

"It's definitely something I have thought about doing in the past, but I just wasn't sure that I'd have the confidence to pose in a bikini on stage in front of an audience of people I don't know," I laughed.

"Yes, it's definitely not for everyone, but I'll introduce you to my old bodybuilding coach, and he can explain the entire process to you. You can ask him anything you want to know."

I felt a fire in my belly suddenly ignite when I realised that this was something I knew I could excel in with minimal changes to my current routine. A week later, I'd paid a five-hundred-dollar deposit and committed myself to a new fitness journey that I was incredibly excited about.

* * * * *

I walked upstairs and followed my new coach into the small consultation room that was tucked away in the corner of the gym and sat on the office chair that he had prepared for me. My eyes were immediately drawn to the forms and paperwork he had laid out on his desk in front of us as he proceeded to explain the entire process that I would be following over the next four months: my new five-day a week gym program, a well-thought-out nutrition plan, the posing practise schedule, regular weigh-ins and photo comparisons to track my progress. As I listened to him ramble off the many components required to bring a unique, well-proportioned and muscular physique to the stage, I began to feel a little on edge about how strict everything was starting to sound.

"I will be keeping track of your body weight, your body fat percentage and your circumference measurements on a regular basis, and we will have weekly check-ins to monitor your progress," my coach explained.

He motioned me to stand in front of him so that he could take all of my circumference measurements with a plastic tape measure: my thighs, the widest part of my bottom, the smallest part of my stomach, my arms and my chest.

I was excited to see my body change, to build the physique of my dreams, but deep down, I knew that the structure and rigidity around calorie intake and training routines were more intense than what I'd ever put myself through. I could feel myself starting to doubt my decision to commit to something that I had essentially worked so hard to move away from.

At this time, I was working as a strength and conditioning sports performance coach, where the training sessions were aimed at improving the athlete's strength, power, speed and agility required for their specific sport. Although I now had a goal to work towards, I couldn't help but feel a little embarrassed when I told my colleagues that I was essentially preparing to be critiqued on my physical appearance.

* * * * *

I had completed two weeks of my new training program, stuck to my meal plan, and had been to two posing practice sessions, which made me realise how incredibly difficult it was to stand in the correct position and then transition from one pose to the next in order to effectively showcase my physique. All I knew was that I felt terribly awkward, and my posing needed a significant amount of work.

Something about this new body-building commitment just didn't feel quite right. My mind was screaming at me to pull out, and my heart was telling me that there was something else out there for me. I just needed to keep searching. I sat on my bed, running through all the possible scenarios in my head before breaking down in a panic, feeling ashamed and disappointed in myself for wanting to quit. I didn't want to let anyone down or be seen as a failure, but I knew that my mental and physical health was more important than trying to pursue something that wasn't wholeheartedly fulfilling me.

I decided to send my coach a text to explain, and the immediate flood of relief I experienced was perfect confirmation that I had made the right decision.

"Decide what you want. Believe you can have it.
Believe you deserve it and believe it's possible for you."

– Jack Canfield

28

I'd recently started to become more intrigued by the idea of manifestation, the law of attraction and visualisation – being able to use the power of the mind to create the reality I wanted to experience. I'd personally never consciously manifested anything in my life before, and I was still a little sceptical about how the whole process worked. I knew it wasn't as easy as simply thinking about manifesting one thousand dollars and watching it land in my bank account the following day. I knew that manifestation required intentional effort, a positive mindset and consistent action towards my goals, but I was willing to give it a go.

I decided to create a vision board filled with images, quotes and symbols of all the things that I wanted to achieve in the near or distant future – one of which was my dream car at the time. I sat this board on my desk so that I could look at it every day and be reminded of my current aspirations and the endless possibilities that this world had to offer.

* * * * *

I was on my way to my local station to catch the train to uni for an anatomy exam I had that morning, and I was meeting Sam at the next stop.

I had my music playing through my doggy aux cord as I drove through the lanes in the parking lot, keeping my eyes peeled for the closest vacant car park.

All of a sudden, out of the corner of my eye, I saw a small red Holden heading straight through the double-empty car park directly perpendicular to me at a rather fast speed. He gave himself no time to stop before forcefully colliding into the front left side of me.

My heart leapt into my throat.

"What the fuck!" I yelled as I stalled my car abruptly and sat there with my hands gripped tightly onto the steering wheel in shock.

I looked over to see a young male driver, who was only on his provisional licence, sitting in his car with a horrified look on his face. We got out of our vehicles and nervously walked around to see the damage.

"I'm so sorry! I was in a rush to catch the train," he blurted out as if that was some kind of excuse to be driving so recklessly through a car park.

"Yeah. So am I," I said bluntly, looking at my now half-attached front bumper and then noticing that the front of his car had nothing but a few scratches.

Typical.

"Just let me park, and then I'll get your number," I said in a hurry, mindful of the fact that my train was coming in less than five minutes.

I quickly got back into my car, unsure if it was safe to drive but knowing I couldn't just leave it in the middle of the lane. There was an empty car park about fifty metres ahead of me.

Perfect.

I turned on the engine, put it into first gear and slowly released the clutch as the car started to move forward. I could hear the bumper scraping against the gravel road and something else rubbing against my front left tyre. Whatever it was, it didn't sound good. The guy walked over to me and gave me his full name and number.

"Again, I'm so sorry. I know it was my fault," he admitted.

"It's okay," I said, forgivingly. "I'll contact my insurance company and be in touch."

He nodded, and we awkwardly began to walk in the same direction.

My station was one of the first stops along our fifty-minute journey, which meant I could usually get Sam and me a double seat next to each other before they all filled up. I sent Sam a message to let him know what carriage to get on and kept my eye out for him as he stepped onto the train. When he sat down next to me, my eyes instantly started to well with tears as I explained to him what had just happened.

"Did you get any photos? His licence plate or any details about his insurance company?" he asked. I didn't have a positive answer to any of his questions.

"No. I didn't even think about any of that. I was so focused on not missing my train because of my exam," I told him, feeling completely stupid that I hadn't got any of this vital information.

"Eb, you need those details! This guy could literally turn this around and blame you for the damage."

"Shit. I'm such an idiot," I replied, putting my head in my hands in frustration.

"I'll get off at the next stop and go back. Tell me what car it was and roughly where you've parked. I'll find it and take photos," he offered generously.

"Sam, you don't have to do that. It's my mistake, I'll deal with it. He seemed really genuine about it. I'm sure it will be fine," I said, trying to convince him.

"You put too much trust in people you don't know, Eb. Who knows what his parents will say to him," he fought back.

I knew I'd really messed up, and I felt terrible about making Sam pick up the pieces for me.

"Thank you. You are too good to me," I said as I gave him a warm hug of appreciation.

Unfortunately, or maybe fortunately, after four fruitful years of driving around my good ol' Swifty, she ended up being a write off. My insurance company gave me a payout for more than I was expecting to sell it for, which meant that the car I had been manifesting for over a year to gift myself for my twenty-first birthday came early. Maggie, the Mazda, had become the newest member of the family. Sometimes, things really do work out in your favour.

"People think a soul mate is your perfect fit, and that's what everyone wants. But a true soul mate is a mirror, the person who shows you everything that is holding you back, the person who brings you to your attention so you can change your life."

– Elizabeth Gilbert

29

Sam and I were walking through the shopping centre, searching for a place to eat for lunch while having a rather in-depth conversation about my anxiety around food.

"I wish I could just eat like everyone else, without thinking about the calories and overanalysing every ingredient in every meal." I clenched my fists and looked up to the ceiling in frustration as I proceeded to think about where I wanted to go for lunch that wasn't going to spike my anxiety.

As we stepped onto the escalator that was heading down towards the outdoor area, I suddenly felt a compelling urge to share with him a secret I'd been too ashamed to share with anyone for months now.

"Sam, there's something that I want to tell you about. Something that I do occasionally that I know probably isn't a good thing." I looked down at my feet to avoid making eye contact with him.

"What do you mean? What is it?" Concern suddenly filled the tone behind his voice.

I knew I'd just opened a large can of worms that I wasn't sure I was quite ready to set free, and I instantly regretted my decision to open my mouth.

"Ah, I wish I didn't say anything. It's so silly," I said as I tried to back out, knowing full well that he wasn't going to let me.

He grabbed my arm to stop me from walking forward and spun me around so that I was forced to look directly at him.

"What is it, Eb? You can't say that and then not tell me."

Dammit.

He was right. I had to tell him now, and although part of me wanted to, I was almost too embarrassed to expose this part of myself that no one yet knew.

I took a deep breath in.

"Well, sometimes, when I see something that I really want to eat, something that I'm craving, like a cookie or a pastry, I'll shove the whole thing in my mouth, chew it until I'm about to swallow and then spit it out."

Okay, there, I said it.

"Eb…," he paused. "Why do you do that?" His tone was now soft and tender as he looked at me with such compassion in his eyes.

"I know it's silly, but when I do it, it's like I get the satisfaction of eating the thing I really want without actually ingesting the calories," I tried to explain myself so that it didn't sound so ridiculous.

"When did you start doing that?" he asked.

"A while ago. But to be honest, I didn't even realise what I was doing when it first started. It was only recently when I started to do it more often, I had this sudden realisation that it's sort of one step away from having bulimia, just without swallowing the food and throwing it back up." It was hard to admit this to him and myself, but it was the truth, a truth that, quite frankly, scared me a little.

"Eb, that's not good. I wish you told me about this sooner. Please promise me you won't do it anymore."

I wanted to promise him that I would stop, but a part of me didn't want to. I had essentially figured out a way to enjoy the taste of the food that I would never allow myself to eat without the feeling of guilt afterwards. But deep down, I knew that this mentality was unhealthy. It needed to change, and now I had Sam to hold me accountable.

"Yes, I will stop," I told him.

* * * * *

Three and a half years had passed by, and our relationship continued to be full of wonderful adventures together. We travelled to Vietnam and went skydiving over the picturesque ocean in Airlie Beach. Sam planned an incredible party at his work venue for my twenty-first birthday, and I surprised him with a second trip to Hamilton Island for his.

We were at the point in our relationship where we both felt ready to take the next step and move in together. It just so happened that around this same time, Aunty Jan and Rex had been thinking about putting their old house up for rent, and Sam and I were the perfect candidates. It couldn't have been more convenient for me; I didn't have to move very far. Sam and I were so excited to finally have our own space and build the life we wanted to live as a couple.

With that came many conversations about marriage, what style of ring I wanted, what our price range was for buying a house, and how many children we wanted to have – we were in it for the long haul.

* * * * *

Moving in together came with its own set of challenges, a new list of responsibilities that we quickly had to learn how to navigate and overcome, but it didn't take us long to get into the groove of things and find our way of doing things.

It was like a breath of fresh air when I came to realise just how much freedom came with living out of home, and I thrived off being the queen of the house. I weirdly got excited about doing my grocery shopping, to finally be able to cook what I wanted, when I wanted and how I wanted. I had more control over my life than I'd ever had before, and it was invigorating.

Sam knew that my type A personality liked things to be done in a certain way, which meant that he'd leave me to my own devices and let me be in charge of the domestic chores – I guess it was easier that way. I had created a weekly routine; I did all the shopping and the cleaning on a Saturday or Sunday morning, as well as all the meal prep for our lunches for the following week.

As the months went by and the novelty of it all began to wear thin, I couldn't help but start to feel like a housewife, dreading having to do the weekly chores, and I knew this was not how I wanted my life to be.

The thing was, I didn't have to clean the house every single weekend, I didn't have to meal prep Sam's lunches, I knew he was more than capable of doing it for himself, but being the overly regimented and pedantic person that I was, I had put the pressure on myself to uphold some kind of standard that I had initially set, without realising that the control I needed to have over my own life, was beginning to interfere with the way Sam lived his.

We had been living together for just over twelve months, and cracks were beginning to form. We had stopped going out on random date nights unless it was a special occasion, mostly because our weekends were dedicated to work or study, and I felt that our relationship was beginning to feel a little stale.

With my number one love language being acts of service, I began to notice myself doing all the little things for Sam that I so desperately wanted him to do for me. I would surprise him with a cooked breakfast on a Sunday morning, buy him his favourite chocolate while I was at the supermarket, bring him a coffee while he was studying or working in the office, and always made sure dinner was ready for him when he arrived home from work. I just wanted him to show me that he loved me in the ways that would fill up my cup too.

Although I communicated this to him, I wrote him letters to express my feelings, and we had a number of serious conversations about how we could bring the spark back to our relationship – he even went to stay with his dad for a week to give me the space I thought I needed – it didn't take long for the same problems to resurface soon after.

'The grass isn't always greener on the other side, Eb,' he'd say, trying to convince me that what we had was worth fighting for. But I wasn't necessarily looking for greener grass. I didn't want to end our relationship so that I could find someone better. I knew the love I had for him was like no other love I had ever experienced before – he meant the absolute world to me, and I know I meant the same to him. But he had been my first and only love, and the little voice deep inside of me was beginning to get louder, making me question what it was that I really wanted from all of this.

For the last five years, Sam had been my rock in every sense of the word. He had helped me to become a better version of myself in so many ways. He showed me that there was so much more to life than spending all my time and energy worrying about every penny I spent or every calorie I put into my mouth. That putting myself first was often more important than trying to please everyone else. He taught me how to live life a little less seriously and just let go. And for that, I was incredibly grateful.

But I started to realise how much I relied on him for my happiness and that I didn't really know how to be truly content within myself without having him by my side. I needed to learn how to be my own support system, how to be totally okay being on my own, without relying on anyone else to pick up the pieces for me.

The thought of ending our relationship made me feel sick to the stomach. I couldn't bear the thought of hurting him, and I wasn't sure if it was the right decision. But I had come to the realisation that in the midst of trying to improve our relationship, I was beginning to lose more of myself in the process.

"Every ray of sunshine, every drop of rain,
every tear that falls, you are with me
for I carry you in my heart forever."

– Heather Wolf

30

I was on the phone with Aunty Jan when she said she had something that she needed to tell me.

"Ebonie, Bella had a nasty fall today and has hurt her dodgy knee quite badly. As she was running around the house this morning, she slipped and fell off the ledge of the decking. It looked like she'd broken it or torn a ligament. She wasn't putting any of her weight on it at all. I took her straight to the vet this afternoon so that he could assess the damage, and I'm sorry, Ebonie, I wish I had better news."

My chest suddenly tightened, and I wasn't sure if I wanted to hear what was coming next. She'd been to visit our local vet on a fairly regular basis over the last couple of years about this particular leg after we noticed her walking with a slight limp that seemed to be getting worse. She was then diagnosed with arthritis, and we were told there wasn't much that we could do other than give her daily medication to help ease her discomfort.

"Adam told me that Bella's leg is basically unrecoverable. She would need to have significant surgery to completely remove her leg, but given that she's already nine, he has recommended that she be put down. I'm so sorry."

Her tone was soft and gentle. The expression completely fell from my face, and my heart dropped to the floor at the thought of having to say goodbye to my baby.

On her last evening with us, I made her a dog-friendly – not that it mattered all that much – apple cake that she devoured in seconds before looking up at me as if to say, 'More?'

It had only been a few days since we'd found out the devastating news, and I was still struggling to imagine a life without my Bella in it. She would no longer be waiting for me at the front door, wagging her tail with pure happiness when she saw me walking towards her. I would no longer be able to gently blow on her ears and laugh as I watched her try to catch the puffs of air like she was trying to catch flies. There would be no more nighttime cuddles when she was in her most docile state of being or watching her twitch and muffle a woof while she was dreaming in her sleep. The bundle of joy that my mum had brought into my life, the unconditional love and affection that she gave me each and every day, was about to come to an end.

* * * * *

Aunty Jan, Sam and I were all sitting outside our local veterinary surgery with Bella girl lying at our feet after being given a sedative to make her sleepy, blissfully unaware that these were going to be her last moments with us.

When we lifted her onto the clinic table, I buried my face into the side of her not so jet black but rather grey muzzle and wrapped my arms around her warm, calm body for the very last time, tears welling in my eyes.

After a few moments, I took a step back and nodded my head at Adam to indicate that I was ready.

"She won't feel a thing," he whispered as he injected the second medication into the vein in her back leg.

I looked into her sad, sleepy eyes and watched as she slowly slipped away.

"Find the thing that makes you passionate and do that… in the end, the things that give the most fulfilment are the things you do for others."

– Tony Blair

31

I was at the end of the third year of my degree and had decided to play it smart and do my compulsory placements throughout the summer semester, which meant that I could have a slightly lighter subject load in my final year.

The clinical placements were separated into two six-week blocks at two different exercise physiology clinics of our preference.

After having to drive a fair way to reach my first block of placement, always planning to account for the ridiculous amount of peak-hour traffic on the roads, I was thrilled to have received my second six-week block at a private clinic that was much closer to home; a neurological rehabilitation centre that provides services to people who had a spinal cord injury, traumatic brain injury, stroke, multiple sclerosis, cerebral palsy and a range of other conditions. It was a very niche field within the realm of exercise physiology that I had not yet had any experience with.

As I walked through the purple doors on my very first day, thirty minutes before client sessions began, wearing my navy blue uni polo shirt and standard black gym tights, I was eagerly welcomed by one of the big bosses, who had just finished a heavy set of bench presses. He slid himself up from under the bar and began walking in my direction. As he got closer, he held out his arm to introduce himself.

"G'day mate, I'm Jim."

"Hi, I'm Ebonie. Nice to meet you," my hand swiftly met his, and he gave it a firm shake.

"Nice to meet you, Grace," he looked at me with the goofiest grin smeared across his face as I tilted my head to the side in confusion.

That's not what I said, but okay… I thought to myself.

I let out a little giggle as our hands disconnected, and he proceeded to show me towards the office, where the rest of the team was piling in as they arrived for the day.

I later found out that Jim never calls the new placement students by their actual names; everyone is given a nickname for no particular rhyme or reason. Whatever shoots to his mind at that very moment is the name that was there to stay, and mine was Grace. From that day on, I knew I was going to love this place.

It wasn't just the fun, bubbly and witty crew that made my work experience so memorable, but also the incredibly motivated, inspirational and strong-willed clients who I got to work with every day, the people who unintentionally opened my eyes to the simple things in life that I too often took for granted; the people who helped me to leave work feeling a little more grateful than I had been the day before.

* * * * *

My six-week placement came to an end, and I had already decided that this was now my dream job; this was where I wanted to spend my time, doing what I loved, helping some of the most incredible people. Unfortunately, they weren't in a position to hire any new trainers, so instead, I offered to volunteer a couple of days a week, secretly hoping that if a position did become available, I'd be the next in line.

Once again, I began to manifest this dream to become my reality. I journaled about it, visualised it, and imagined myself wearing a purple shirt and being a part of the team. I told myself that my time would come; I just needed to continue showing up, putting in the effort, and being patient.

It was my second day of volunteering, and I was in the massage room folding the towels, ready for the day ahead, when Jim suddenly poked his head around the corner and started chatting to me about how my study was going and how much longer I had left of my course.

"Yeah, cool. So, we'd like to offer you a job," he slid in a very important piece of information as casually as you could imagine.

I dropped the towel onto the massage bed and immediately turned my head to look at him.

"No way!" I gasped, cupping my hands over my mouth that had already dropped to the floor, the happy tears beginning to well in my eyes.

"Yep," he said, clearly thrilled by how excited I was.

"I can't believe it!" I was the most excited I'd been in a long time; I even hugged him.

"Thank you so much. You have no idea how much this means to me."

I was now officially a part of the purple family.

I was hired to work as an assistant for the next ten months until

I finished my degree and was then able to take sessions without supervision.

As an exercise physiologist, I knew that I could help an athlete jump a little higher, run a little faster or throw a little further; it could be the difference between them winning or losing their major event.

But knowing I also had the potential to help people regain their ability to take independent steps, transfer in and out of a car, bring a spoon to their mouth or hold their child in their arms, this meant so much more to me than helping someone to win a race ever would. The clients became more than just clients; some of them became dear friends and I thank my lucky stars to have crossed paths with them in this lifetime.

"Letting someone go doesn't always mean that you don't love them anymore. It means that you love yourself enough to become the person you need to be without them."

– Charlotte Freeman

32

I had finished work for the afternoon, and my colleague, Tim, who had also become one of my closest friends since I started working at Making Strides, could tell that I had not been my normal bubbly, chatty self.

"Eb, are you okay? You seem a bit off today," he offered his concern.

"Not really," I replied, looking down at my feet, trying desperately not to burst into tears in front of him. There's something about someone asking you if you're okay that makes you suddenly feel like you're even worse than you thought.

"Do you want to go for a drive and talk about it?" Tim had been with his partner at the time for almost eight years, so I knew that if there were anyone who'd be able to understand some of what I was feeling, it would be him.

"Yes, I'd really like that," I said softly as I felt a wave of relief wash over me, hoping that he might be able to help make my head feel a little clearer.

We arrived at North Burleigh Beach, a short ten-minute drive from our workplace, and found a quiet spot on the sand to sit and watch as the colours in the sky changed from orange to pink to purple while the sun went down for another evening.

"I don't know what to do, Tim. I feel like my heart knows what it wants, but my head is trying to pull me in the opposite direction." I felt my eyes begin to well with the tears that I'd been holding back the entire day.

"I love him so much, but I'm not sure if I'm in love with him anymore. I keep trying to convince myself that I am, that he is everything I want, but I don't think I even know what it is that I want. I feel like I have this burning desire to break free and experience life on my own for a little while." I closed my eyes and let the tears fall down my cheeks.

"I feel like such a terrible person; he doesn't deserve this."

He put his arm around my shoulders and pulled me in towards him.

"Eb, you can't beat yourself up for how you feel. You have to do what is right for you, and sometimes you have to be a little selfish."

"I know. But how do I do that when I know how much I'm going to hurt him? It honestly feels like my heart is being ripped to pieces, knowing that I'm going to break his." I looked up towards the sky and took a deep breath in, hoping that the tears might sink back into the back of my eyeballs.

"The thought of going from sharing every single part of myself with one person for the last five years to nothing at all scares me so much," I looked back at Tim, my eyes full of fear.

"What if I don't ever find anyone else who loves me as much as he does? What if I ruin the only good thing that's ever happened to me?"

"It's never an easy decision, Eb, but sometimes you have to let someone go in order to realise who you are without them."

We talked for what felt like hours, and by the end of our conversation, I finally had some clarity. I knew what I needed to do.

* * * * *

I bawled my eyes out the entire drive home before pulling into my driveway and contemplating my life for another ten minutes in the car. When Sam arrived home from work, I had dinner prepared and ready for him on the table. I had already eaten mine, but I sat across from him while he ate in silence. He could tell something wasn't right.

"I don't think I can do this anymore," I eventually blurted out, tension radiating from every word.

He finished his mouthful of food and looked up at me; the expression fell from his face.

"Do what?"

I felt terrible. I hated every minute of this conversation, but I knew I couldn't wait any longer.

"This. Us. I think I need to be on my own for a while."

He didn't seem shocked at all. It was like he knew exactly what was coming. He dropped his gaze away from mine and looked down at his plate of food, nodding his head slowly in complete despair.

"Okay."

He didn't try to fight it; he knew that this was what I wanted, and he chose to accept it.

* * * * *

After I'd had my shower, I walked into the office to check on him.

"Sammy, are you okay?" He spun around on his desk chair to see me standing in front of him, and I realised from his red and puffy eyes that he'd obviously been crying. I sat down next to him on the hard wooden floorboards with my back leaning up against the wall behind me.

"I really am so sorry." My eyes began to well.

"Please just know that I need to do this for myself. I know that if we're meant to be together, we will be." I blubbered my way through, trying to reassure him as the tears continued to stream down my cheeks.

"No, Eb, you know I don't believe in that. If you're ending it now, this is it. I know it is."

He quickly rubbed his fingers across his eyes to wipe away his tears. Sam never believed in the universal 'everything happens for a reason' logic that I did, so this wasn't reassuring for him. We spent one last night together, crying, laughing a little, before crying some more, and strangely enough, I felt more connected to him that evening than I had in a while.

* * * * *

The moment my eyes opened the following morning, the tears began to spill over, falling down my cheeks like a river escaping a dam. Although it had all been my decision, it felt like I had just been stabbed with a knife in the chest, and I was struggling to ease the pain. Ending the relationship was one of the scariest and most difficult decisions I had ever had to make, and I still felt incredibly torn as to whether I had made the right decision or not. But it was the immense guilt I felt for leaving him that was almost enough to make me want to stay, and I knew I couldn't do that to either of us.

As I watched him pack up everything he owned and shove it into the bags that he had lying on the bed, I knew I had to get out of there before I changed my mind.

I got into my car, my hands shaking as I gripped tightly onto the steering wheel with absolutely no idea of where I was going. Within five minutes, I had decided to drive to my very close family friend Maddie's house. Maddie had known me for almost my entire life. I treated her like another mum, and I knew I could count on her to be there for me.

The moment she opened her front door to let me in, the waterworks had begun. I fell into her arms, letting her take the weight of my body as I sobbed over her shoulder, and an involuntary whimper escaped from my lips.

"Oh, Eb. What happened?" She ran her hands through my hair and pulled it back behind my ears, away from my weeping eyes.

"I ended things with Sam," I told her, wiping away the teardrops from under my nose.

"Come sit on my bed. I'll run you a hot bath, and you can tell me everything."

* * * * *

I stayed with Maddie that night. I hadn't spoken to Sam since I'd left the house, and I was already missing having him by my side. I suddenly felt so alone. Every time I closed my eyes, my heart felt like it was going to explode. Fear began to shoot through me as I tried to swallow back the panic that threatened to creep up my throat. The only person I wanted, the only person who I knew would make me feel any calmer, was him.

I quietly crept out of the bedroom, trying not to wake Maddie, who was asleep beside me. I knew it was a bad idea, but I just needed to hear his voice. I dialled his number and waited anxiously for him to answer.

The ringing stopped, "Sam?" I waited for him to say something.

"Eb, what's wrong?"

"I don't know, but I don't feel good. I can't sleep, and I feel so sick. I feel like I'm having a panic attack. I'm so sorry for doing this. I'm so sorry for hurting you." I didn't know what I was saying but I just wanted him to know how much I was hurting, too, how guilty I was feeling.

"Eb, it's fine. Don't worry about me." Silence filled the air, neither of us wanting to say anything.

"I don't know what else to say," he said finally. His voice sounded so broken, and I just wanted to do anything I could to make it better.

"Please know that you will always hold a special place in my heart. I will always love you," I confessed, unsure if that was the right thing to say.

"I know, Eb. So will you."

I got off the phone and laid on the couch in the living room, cuddling a pillow firmly against my chest, trying to cling onto anything that gave me some form of comfort. I let the floodgates open once again and allowed the emotions to break free. It was one of the most difficult nights I'd ever experienced.

"Anything that gets your blood racing is probably worth doing."

– Hunter S. Thompson

33

I ended up moving in with Maddie after Sam and I went our separate ways. I decided I couldn't live in the old cottage anymore; it was the house I'd moved into after Mum died, it was where I'd spent most of my time with Bella, and it was where Sam and I had started building our future together – too many memories that I knew were not going to help me move on. Maddie's unit was in the perfect location – it was closer to the beach, closer to my work and closer to most of my friends. Something about her place felt so homely; I felt safe, comfortable and free to be me. I knew it was the fresh start I needed.

I decided to join a new gym located just around the corner, where I met a personal trainer, who later became one of my best mates, and after a few months, he introduced me to the sport of olympic weightlifting. At first, it was just a bit of fun. I had never intended on taking it too seriously, but for the first time in years, my training was far less centred around how I looked, and more on how I was performing. My olympic lifting technique was embarrassingly atrocious, but I was so eager to learn these new skills. Luckily, Lach was patient enough to teach me the basics of each lift and kind enough to write me a training program to help put it into practice.

After a couple of months, I started to realise how much I enjoyed this style of training, and I knew that this was very much a sport that I could one day compete in, a sport that I could actually commit to and excel in if I put in the effort. I decided to reach out to my old personal trainer, who had competed in many weightlifting competitions himself and had recently started offering group strength and olympic weightlifting classes to his clients. He was stoked to have me back on board his team.

Towards the end of 2021, I took part in my first in-house weightlifting competition. Although it wasn't official, it allowed me to experience the thrill and satisfaction of completing a successful lift on the platform in front of a proper audience. From that day forward, I was obsessed. I had finally found a sport that lit up my soul and made me hungry for more.

After my first official competition in December of 2021, I decided that I wanted to try qualifying for the 2022 Queensland state championships. It wasn't going to be easy, but I was determined to make it happen.

I needed a combined lifting total of one-hundred and twenty-two kilograms, which meant that I had eight months to build an extra twenty-two kilograms onto my lifts... somehow. I bought myself a one-piece weightlifting suit, some knee sleeves, a weightlifting belt, and a more legit pair of weightlifting shoes. The outfit was absolutely a necessary piece of the puzzle.

On the day of my third-ever competition, I was feeling a bit under the weather. I had been struck with a dreadful head cold a few days prior, which meant that I'd missed my last few days of training, and this made me feel even more nervous than I already was. I was relying significantly on the rush of adrenalin I knew I'd get as I stepped up onto the platform to magically make the weight fly above my head.

I was stoked to have completed all six of my lifting attempts, but unfortunately, I hadn't qualified for states this time round.

I was standing amongst the crowd watching the others complete their lifts, with Lach and my other mate Max who had come to support me. After a few moments, I noticed one of the spectators walking towards me with a concerned look on her face. "Ebonie, I'm sorry, we have just realised that we made a calculation error, and you actually lifted the same weight for your final two attempts in the clean and jerk. We are happy to give you another attempt at a heavier weight if you'd like?"

My heart fluttered with excitement at the thought of having another chance. I looked over at Lach.

"Should I do it?" I asked.

"Absolutely! Let's go get you warmed up again." He nudged me on the arm, and I followed him outside.

I was about halfway through my warmup reps when she came out to see me again, "You only have to lift an extra four kilos to qualify for states. I know it's a big jump, but you have nothing to lose, so I reckon you should go for it."

"Okay, let's do it!" I replied immediately before realising that I had just committed to a seventy-kilogram clean and jerk that I'd never lifted before.

I was the final lifter of the day, and as I walked up to the platform, my coach, who was also running the competition, announced to the audience,

"This is a qualifying lift for Ebonie and will also be a personal best."

No pressure.

The crowd cheered and clapped as I prepared myself for what I knew was going to be extremely heavy.

I gave myself a few moments to set up my foot position before squatting down to wrap my hands tightly around the bar. I closed my eyes and took a deep breath in, before looking up to the room full of people staring at me in complete silence. I locked my eyes on a single spot in front of me, and then I went for it. I yanked the bar off the ground with everything I had and managed to catch the clean.

Man, that felt heavy, I thought.

I stood there for what felt like the longest time, my entire body shaking and my heart pounding through my chest as I prepared myself for the next and hardest part of the lift.

"Take a breather," my coach called out.

"Yes! Come on, Eb, you've got this!" Lach shouted at me. I counted down, three, two, one… before aggressively punching the bar above my head and letting out a cheeky grin when I felt my elbows lock, and I knew that I had secured the lift. I waited for the signal from my coach before dropping the bar to the ground. I put my hands together and smiled from ear to ear with excitement. I had just qualified for states.

* * * * *

I had six months until the big event, with another local competition in two months, so I knew I had plenty of time to build up my numbers and smash some goals.

I had never trained so intensely in my life, and my body absolutely knew about it. My thighs were always bruised from the impact of the bar bouncing off my legs, my shins often took a beating as I lifted the bar from the ground, trying to keep it close, scraping the skin away, and the muscles in my neck were always wound up from the weight I'd be lifting above my head, but none of this stopped me. I was in the gym at half past five in the morning four days a week, following my coach's lifting program to a tee, always hoping to see a little bit of progress. Every time I hit a new personal best, the fire in my belly would reignite and only make me hungry for more.

But of course, as the weight of my lifts continued to increase, my body weight did, too, and I was beginning to notice how much muscle bulk I had gained over the last twelve months. Although my weight was sitting at its heaviest, I was the strongest, fittest and healthiest I'd ever felt. My menstrual cycle was back, which meant my hormones were finally starting to regulate. People around me began to comment on how strong I was looking and how impressed they were with the weight I was lifting, compliments that I very much appreciated. I knew that if I wanted to be a successful weightlifter and achieve the goals that I had set for myself, I needed to be okay with putting on a few extra kilos. I couldn't build the strength that I needed and be as lean as I wanted all at the same time; that's just not how the system worked. But it was a constant battle in my head, one that was starting to get harder to fight against.

I stood in front of the mirror, once again, picking myself apart. My legs were noticeably thicker, my clothes were getting tighter, and I could feel the confidence I had in my body that I had worked so hard for beginning to take a downward spiral… again. Competing in states was the one thing getting me through.

* * * * *

Having the opportunity to compete in the Queensland State Championships for Olympic weightlifting was truly one of my greatest achievements, an event that I was incredibly proud to be part of.

My lifting time wasn't until five o'clock in the afternoon, which wasn't my preferred time of day to be lifting, and it also meant that I had the entire day to wallow in the pit of nerves sitting at the bottom of my stomach. I arrived at the facility a couple of hours early to get myself prepared for my big event, and the first thing I noticed was how official everything was. The lifting platform was huge, much bigger than I'd seen before. The entire competition was live-streamed, and all the competitors were given an identification number to pin onto their suits.

I said hello to my coach, who had been there all day, and he directed me out the back to where there were about eight other warm-up platforms. I put my bags down and made my way to the lady's bathroom to complete my weigh-in. I knew that I had nothing to worry about. I was well within the seventy-one-kilo weight class, but there was always the little voice in the back of my head that made me doubt my confidence.

I pushed the door open to see the two ladies standing with their clipboards, ticking everyone off their list as they came through. I gave them my name and removed my sandals and my jumper so that I was left standing in my one-piece suit, ready to step onto the scales.

One of the girls put her hand out to stop me.

"You will need to take everything off before we take your weight," she ordered.

She wants me to get naked?

My brows furrowed, confused.

"Everything?" I asked.

She could tell I clearly hadn't done this before.

"Yes, sorry," she replied.

Thankfully, they only let one person in the room at a time, so it wasn't like I was stripping off nude in front of a group of people. I timidly removed my suit and my underwear and stepped onto the scales, feeling extremely vulnerable as I stood there looking down at the number. Just over sixty-eight kilograms, perfect. As soon as they recorded the number, I swiftly put my clothes back on and got the heck out of there.

The level of nervousness I felt as I walked onto the platform was unlike any other competition I'd ever done before. My entire body was shaking before I'd even lifted any weight. I had my mini support crew sitting in the audience, cheering me on amongst a bunch of strangers, and because I was one of the weakest competitors in my weight class, I was the second lifter in my section.

Again, no pressure.

My heart sunk to the floor when I thought I'd caught the bar at the bottom of my snatch but couldn't quite hold it, dropping it in front of me for the second time at a weight that I had completed hundreds of times before. I walked off the platform feeling completely defeated, knowing that if I failed my next attempt, I would be out of the competition completely.

Every part of me wanted to give up, to pack my bags and go home. But I had not worked this hard to give up so easily. That's not the person I wanted to be. I had to get my head back in the game.

My dear friend Georgia, who had come to support me, followed me into the bathroom, where she found me shedding the tears I was trying so hard to hold in. Georgia was also an Olympic weightlifter but had been doing it for a lot longer than I had, which meant she had a lot more experience under her belt and had been in my position many times before. Her pep talk was exactly what I needed to hear, and I felt so grateful to have her there with me.

"You need to get angry! Get out there and be aggressive. You know you've got this!" She gave me a cheeky slap on the booty and then wrapped her arms around my waist to give me a tight squeeze.

When I walked back out onto the platform, exuding as much confidence as I could muster up, I pulled the forty-eight-kilogram bar so hard off the floor and managed to successfully catch my third and final snatch attempt.

Phew.

It wasn't the weight I was aiming for, but I'd done it. I was back in.

I had just nailed my first two clean-and-jerk attempts, matching my current personal best of seventy-six kilos, and I was now onto my third lift for the evening.

I walked back onto the platform for the final time, trying to control my breathing as my heart was thumping through my chest and my hands jittered as I reached down to hook grip the bar. This was it; I knew I had it in me. It was just a matter of how badly I wanted it. I closed my eyes, took a deep breath in, and did what Georgia had told me to do. I got angry.

I ripped the bar from the ground and caught the clean at the bottom, tensing every muscle in my body to help me stand up from the deep squat I'd landed in. The adrenaline was pumping through my veins as I now prepared myself to punch the eighty-kilogram bar over my head.

Before I knew it, the bar was directly above me, my elbows had locked, and my support crew, along with the rest of the crowd were cheering as I got the signal to lower the bar to the ground. I couldn't believe I'd actually done it. The feeling was indescribable.

"Don't worry about the speed bumps in the road until you find one that's worth slowing down for."

– James Smith

34

For as long as I can remember, the top of Rex's head was shiny, smooth and very bald. He started losing hair at the ripe age of twenty, and rather than having patches of thin, wispy hair; he decided it was probably more of an attractive look to just shave it all off completely. This meant no hair to protect his scalp from the harsh UV sun rays on a day-to-day basis, and sun safety was also not as prominent back in the seventies or eighties, so his poor head copped a beating.

As he got older and wiser, he clocked on to the importance of wearing a hat while working outdoors, but unfortunately, by his mid-forties, a lot of the damage had already been done. He had routine visits to the doctor to get the spots on his head either burnt off or cut out as a precautionary measure. This became a normal part of his routine.

* * * * *

One morning, as Aunty Jan was helping with his morning routine, she noticed a light pink, shiny-looking bump, the size of a five-cent piece, behind Rex's right ear. This wasn't anything too out of the ordinary for Rex, but they visited the doctor to confirm it wasn't anything serious. She took a biopsy from the slightly raised lump before cutting it out completely, leaving a reasonably deep wound that needed to be stitched and properly taken care of to reduce any risk of infection. The results from the biopsy revealed that it was a basal cell carcinoma (BCC), a very common type of skin cancer that grows slowly and can be easily treated when caught early enough.

Unfortunately, Rex's condition meant that any scrape, cut or damage to the skin took days, weeks, and, in the worst cases, months to completely heal. The wound care nurses came to visit the house every few days to clean and redress the wound, but after a couple of weeks, it didn't seem to be healing as expected; something wasn't quite right. Aunty Jan took Rex back to the doctor, who seemed a little more concerned with its presentation and referred him directly to an Ear, Throat and Nose surgeon for further examination.

After some more tests, the surgeon was finally able to shed some light on what was going on. He revealed that Rex's cancer had grown to the size of a closed fist. He now required immediate surgery, which was then to be followed up by four weeks of radiation therapy to ensure that it was completely gone. Things had just escalated rapidly.

The operation involved removing a significant portion of the right side of Rex's face, including his saliva glands and half of his ear.

Thankfully, Rex's hearing remained intact, but the right side of his mouth now became very dry and sticky due to the lack of saliva production.

When I came to visit Rex after his surgery, he looked more frail than ever. His cheeks were drawn inwards, his shoulders were slumped forward in his chair, and his hands were trembling uncontrollably as he tried to rest them on his legs. My heart broke to see him in such a terrible way. I felt helpless. But no matter how tough it was, Rex continued to keep his chin up, put a smile on his face and soldier on. He was a true fighter.

* * * * *

"Don't forget, Ebonie, you attract what you radiate," he'd remind me every so often.

Rex was a man of very few words, but now and then, he'd allow his sentimental side to shine through and speak words of wisdom.

It was soon after Rex's autoimmune diagnosis that our relationship truly started to blossom. A dear friend once said to me, "If something were to happen to Rex, would you regret not making more of an effort?" My answer at that moment was yes. Deep down, I knew I hadn't been the person I wanted to be. I hadn't shown Rex the appreciation and love that he deserved after adapting so much of his life to fit me into it. He loved me like I was his daughter, and I wanted him to know how grateful I was to have a father figure like him in my life. I owed him that much.

Given that my chosen profession was to work in the neurological space, I offered to visit Rex two or three times a week for an hour or so, specifically to help him with his exercise program. I'd stretch his legs while he was sitting in his chair, we'd do some upper body banded exercises, and then I'd usually finish by giving him a neck massage to help ease his pain.

"I'm just getting weaker every day," he mumbled to me as he tensed all the muscles in his face and struggled to lift the one kilo dumbbell over his head. He then looked up at me with so much fear and disappointment in his eyes. In that moment, I had no words. I could see how terrified he was about what his future looked like, having no control over how it was all going to end. I wanted to encourage him to keep trying to maintain the little strength that he had left, but I didn't know how.

"I can only imagine how hard this must be for you, but you're doing the best you can, and that's all that matters," I said. It was the only thing I could think of that sounded somewhat hopeful.

Those hours together became one of the most thrilling parts of Rex's day. I tried my best to help distract him from his depressive thoughts for as long as I could.

Rex became someone I confided in about many personal things in my life. When I went to visit him, I told him about my highs and lows, my achievements, my failures, my relationships, and my life goals. He sat and listened without any judgment.

"I've been thinking about setting off to travel around Europe. I'd love to actually live somewhere over there for a little while, to experience a new culture, a new lifestyle and use it as an opportunity to see the world."

Rex looked at me sitting across from him, and I noticed a slight change in his eyes. They had suddenly gotten brighter and happier like he was proud of me for even considering such a big change in my life.

"That sounds like a wonderful idea, Ebonie. I think you would regret not going for it," he said.

He was truly my biggest supporter. Nothing was ever too big, nothing was ever too silly, and he only ever encouraged me to chase my dreams.

"You can achieve anything you want, Eb; you've just got to believe in yourself," he smiled softly.

*"It's amazing how someone can break your heart and
you can still love them with all the little pieces."*

– Ella Harper

35

Six years had gone by, and I hadn't heard a single peep from my dad. Not that I was expecting to. I knew that our relationship was over, but for some reason, the same thoughts that I'd had all those years ago were beginning to resurface.

Maybe he's waiting for me to reach out, I thought. Perhaps if I try again, he will respond differently.

Either way, I knew I had nothing to lose, and the little voice deep inside of me was telling me to try one last time.

'Hey Dad, it's me, Eb. I know you probably weren't ever expecting to hear from me again, but you're my dad, and it still hurts not to have anything to do with you. I'm sorry for things that happened in the past, but I'm not a child anymore. I don't want to interfere with your life if it's not something you want, and I will respect any decision you make, but all I ask is that you please read this text and give me the opportunity to talk to you. A phone call or I could see you. Even if it's just once.'

I closed my eyes and felt my heart skip a beat as I quickly sent the message before I changed my mind. I dropped my phone onto the table in front of me and let out a heavy sigh. Even though I knew he probably wouldn't respond, my chest felt a little lighter, like a weight had lifted.

I decided I needed to do something to distract me from the anxious thoughts circulating in my mind, so I got up and started to frantically clean the kitchen.

Thirty minutes later, I heard my phone buzz. I raced over to have a look and couldn't believe my eyes when I saw his name pop up on my screen.

'Hi, Ebonie. I'm sorry, but I made my decision years ago. You hated Julie way back then. I can't see that you would have changed your mind. I'm not prepared to have you come into my life now and try to destroy my relationship with Julie.

I know it was you and your friends ringing us that time. I don't think you have changed. You learnt well from your mother.'

My heart dropped to the floor before shattering into what felt like a million pieces. It was a response, but not the one that I was hoping for.

I had his attention now; I just needed to try harder. I responded within minutes.

'I promise you I won't ever come between you and Julie. That was nearly ten years ago, and I can assure you I've changed. I'm not like my mum. I'm my own person, and I just want you to see that. I will never do anything to jeopardise your relationship. Please trust me. Can I call you just for a few minutes, even if that's all I get?'

I saw the three dots pop up to show he was typing a response.

'No.'

'You won't ever give me another chance?' I quickly typed.

'No.'

'Is there anything I can do?'

'No, Ebonie. Please. You don't need me in your life, and I don't need you. I'm sorry.'

It wasn't a case of me needing him or him needing me. For some stupid reason, I wanted him in my life, but he clearly didn't feel the same. Even after everything, I bowed down to him like he was some divine being and practically begged for his forgiveness.

'But you're my dad. That has to mean something to you. I would honestly do anything. I know I sound fucking desperate, but I'm proud of the person I've become without my parents around. I'm sorry for how I treated you and Julie. It would mean the world for you both to give me a chance.'

I sat by my phone, staying ridiculously hopeful for this man who was supposedly my father to respond with something that I so desperately wanted to read, for him to tell me that he would give me another chance to prove myself to him, but I received nothing. Complete radio silence.

I laid down on the couch, threw my phone to the side and allowed the tears to stream down my cheeks as I tried to comprehend the pure hatred my dad still had towards me.

But I hated him for how much he made my heart ache, how insignificant he made me feel, and how little he cared about me. I clearly meant nothing to him at all, and I couldn't understand why. I cried for hours that afternoon, harder than I'd cried in a long time.

A few hours later, I received another text from him.

'What do you do for work?'

My eyes widened as I felt a sudden flicker of hope race up my spine. He was actually showing some interest in my life.

'I'm an exercise physiologist. I graduated uni at the end of last year. I work mostly with people who have spinal cord injuries.'

'Very good! Have you bought a house?'

Interesting question, but at this point, I was happy with anything.

'Not yet. I have been looking, but the market is not ideal. Are you still working in construction?'

'Yes.'

'Are you still living in the same place?'

'Yes.'

Shit. The short, blunt answers were back, and I immediately started to worry that I'd said the wrong thing.

'Has something changed?' I quickly typed.

'What do you mean?'

'In terms of talking to me?'

'No. Nothing's changed.'

I was so confused. I felt as though I was on a roller coaster and the highs and lows were starting to make my head feel fuzzy.

'Okay. Why did you ask me what I do for work?' I asked

'I didn't. That must have been Norman.'

Who the fuck is Norman?

I couldn't take it anymore. It felt like he was just taking me for a joy ride, laughing to himself behind his phone screen at how pathetic this conversation was.

I decided to leave the conversation for a few hours, running through the thread of messages over and over in my head, trying to figure out what his intentions were but getting absolutely nowhere.

Later that evening, I signed off with a gentle message that I knew would leave the ball in his court.

'Well, thank you for responding. You know where to find me if you ever change your mind. Ebs.'

'I won't ever change my mind, Ebonie! You said that you would respect my decision, so do that!'

His message was loud and clear, and as much as my heart ached, I needed to do what I had promised and leave him alone. I knew it was time to finally let him go.

"Peace: it does not mean to be in a place where there is no noise, trouble or hard work. It means to be in the midst of those things and still be calm in your mind."

– The Secret

36

Rex's health continued to decline. The number of steps he could take before needing to sit down for a rest got smaller and smaller; the amount of assistance required for him to stand out of a chair became greater, and his ability to grip a pen and write a note became weaker. There was a process of grief behind every little function that he lost.

Eventually, Rex's muscles had become so atrophied that he had no choice but to rely on an electric mobility chair to move around the house; he needed to be hoisted from his mobility chair to his bed and required complete assistance when showering or using the toilet. When Rex looked in the mirror, he could barely recognise himself; he was a sixty-five-year-old man in what felt like a one-hundred-year-old person's body.

His body's ability to chew, swallow and digest any form of sustenance properly was also beginning to fail, causing him to develop multiple chest infections, which then led to a diagnosis of aspirated pneumonia and a long-lasting cough that never seemed to completely disappear. After several antibiotic prescriptions and many visits to the hospital, it appeared that the simple act of eating and drinking was causing him more harm than good.

The day that Rex got a feeding tube inserted into his stomach was the day I realised that his condition was completely taking over his body, and there was nothing he or anyone else could do to stop it. It was terrifying. He no longer had the opportunity to enjoy his warm bowl of porridge in the mornings, chew on his favourite pineapple lump lollies, volunteer himself to taste test my homemade treats or sip on his rather flavourless but antioxidant-rich matcha tea. He couldn't even have a drink of water. His daily nutrition now came from a liquid-based formula, full of the essential macronutrients, vitamins and minerals, syringed directly into his stomach four times a day. Any of Rex's medication needed to be crushed and dissolved in water prior to entering the tube, before or after his meal.

He had also recently been diagnosed with moderate sleep apnea and was given a prescription for a CPAP machine, which he quickly opted out of using on most nights. Obviously, this was not the recommended option, but I can only imagine how terribly uncomfortable and disruptive it would be to sleep with a face mask strapped around your head, covering your entire nose and mouth. It was one thing after another. Rex began sleeping on an adjustable mobility bed, and when his coughing became too disruptive to sleep next to, Aunty Jan made the difficult decision to move into the spare room. This was a very sad and unfair realisation that the physical intimacy and romance of their relationship would have to take a back seat.

Twenty-four years ago, Aunty Jan pledged to be Rex's life partner through sickness and in health, and that is exactly what she continued to do as she willingly stepped into the role of being his full-time carer, an adjustment that no one is ever ready for.

* * * * *

Any time Aunty Jan wanted to visit her family in Melbourne for a week or so, she had the overwhelming job of organising twenty-four-hour care for Rex while she was away. She could no longer just book a holiday, pack up a bag and go. She had to meticulously plan out every moment of every day so that she knew she could leave Rex in a safe, comfortable and calm environment without her.

The shifts were separated into day and night, and on one particular occasion, I offered to stay over for a night to help ease the pressure of having to ask one of the carers. My job was to sleep in Aunty Jan's bed with one ear open, listening to the baby monitor she had sitting on her bedside table in case Rex needed some assistance during the night.

It was nine o'clock in the evening, and when I arrived, Rex's carer had already helped him with his nighttime routine, and he was in bed, ready for sleep.

Halfway through the night, as I was tossing and turning, I noticed that Rex had suddenly stopped breathing. I knew this was because of his sleep apnea, so I waited patiently for him to take his next breath. The seconds continued to pass by, and I couldn't hear anything. I started to panic and propped myself up onto one arm, grabbed the baby monitor and listened intently.

Suddenly, Rex took in the biggest gasp of air, as if he'd been startled by someone in his sleep.

Oh, thank goodness, I thought to myself as I let out a huge sigh of relief and laid myself back down.

This breathing pattern continued multiple times throughout the night: loud, rattle-like snoring, followed by thirty seconds of complete silence, which were then interrupted by a sharp inhale of fresh air. It was scary to listen to, and I finally understood what Aunty Jan had to endure every night, something I wasn't sure I'd ever have the strength and patience to cope with.

* * * * *

Rex was admitted to the hospital once again with a chest infection that quickly developed into another spell of pneumonia. He was exhausted. His mind was tired of fighting with everything it had against a body that he felt completely trapped in, with not a single moment of relief. It was all becoming too much, and he was slowly starting to lose his motivation to stay strong.

Aunty Jan sat by Rex's hospital bed, holding his stiff, shaky hand. After being given a cocktail of drugs to help him rest and recover, the coughing finally settled. He lay there quietly, with his eyes closed and his body so still. He was finally in a state of calm. Aunty Jan watched him take his last few breaths as he slowly slipped away as peacefully as he could.

"You can't wait for success to feel empowered.
You can't wait for wealth to feel abundant.
You can't wait for your new relationship to feel loved or
your healing to feel whole. Stop waiting for something
outside of you to change the way you feel on the inside.
Stop giving yourself permission to stay limited."

– Joe Dispenza

37

After Rex had passed, I realised life was too short to be doing the same thing, day in and day out. It felt like I was just rolling through the motions of life with no real direction, no game plan for my future and a serious lack of motivation for anything. Living abroad, particularly in Europe, was something I had dreamt of doing for a long time; the thought of being able to see the world through a different lens and take the opportunity to learn more about myself excited me to my core. I just hadn't had the confidence to make it happen yet, but I was finally ready. I needed a change, and I was hungry for adventure.

It was during my online search for information about living abroad that I stumbled across an agency that promoted working holiday opportunities all over the world. I thought that going through a company like this was the best option for me because it meant that I would be completely guided through the entire process, and it would remove a whole lot of stress on my end.

The experience that stood out to me the most was being able to work as an au pair in a European country with accommodation and meals covered and a small weekly allowance that could go straight towards the travel fund. Having the opportunity to create a home away from home on the other side of the world, becoming a part of a new family, and spending my days off exploring or travelling to a new city, sounded pretty damn good to me.

As I clicked the button to pay the deposit for being an au pair in Italy, I realised that this was probably one of the most spontaneous things I'd ever done. I'd hardly spoken to anyone about this huge decision, which was very unlike me; I just knew it was something I had to do.

The planning began about eight months before I was planning to leave. This gave me a significant amount of time to mentally prepare myself for such a huge change.

Finding a host family was one of the last pieces of the puzzle and, ironically, the one that I wanted to know about most. Living in a foreign, non-English speaking country on the other side of the world was one thing, but moving in with a family of strangers to take on the responsibility of looking after their children was a whole different kettle of fish. I started to get anxious about what kind of family the agency would match me with. I wrote in my journal about what my ideal situation would look like: a family who lived in a perfect location, with easy access to shops and public transport, a family who were somewhat health conscious and understood my passion for health and fitness, and a family that accepted me into their home with open arms.

I had many interviews with a number of families across different parts of Italy, but they continued to fall through for one reason or another.

* * * * *

It was less than two months before I had planned to leave Australia, and I was beginning to feel frustrated and anxious at the thought of not knowing exactly what my plan was, where I was going to be living or who my host family would be. I didn't want to rush the process and end up with a family who I wasn't happy with. I wanted to feel a connection with them from the very first phone call, to find a family that I knew was going to welcome me into a place that I could call home for a while.

I came to realise that something deeper was holding me back from allowing these new and exciting opportunities to enter my life. I needed to temporarily let go of the only place I knew as home, the only place where I had learnt to feel completely safe, secure and content within myself, to create an open space for something else to fill it. I had to allow myself to fully commit to being out of my comfort zone and truly embrace living in the unknown. I needed to trust that the perfect family would enter my life at exactly the right moment.

* * * * *

Just one month prior to jetting off, I got off the phone and raced into Maddie's bedroom, beaming with excitement.

"I've got my host family!" I exclaimed.

They were a family of four with two daughters, aged twelve and seventeen – I would be helping with the younger child. They lived in the North of Italy, directly in the city centre of Turin, with shops at my doorstep and the major train station just around the corner from their house.

Talking to this family and organising everything just felt so effortless; they were the most easy-going family I'd spoken to, more than happy to work around me, with no specific requirements. I connected with them instantly, and I couldn't wait to meet them. They were the perfect family.

I booked my flights two days later. I had a family, a set location and a date of arrival. It was all starting to feel very real.

"Twenty years from now, you will be more disappointed by the things you didn't do than the ones you did."

– Mark Twain

38

After a very long thirty-hour transit, I finally touched down in the fabulous fashion capital of Italy, Milan. It was seven o'clock in the morning, which meant it was five o'clock in the afternoon back at home in Australia. The sleeping tablet I'd taken on my first fourteen-hour long-haul flight had certainly helped to knock me out for most of the journey, but the quality of sleep was not ideal. All I wanted to do was lie horizontal and take a nap, but first, I needed to buy myself a SIM card, take a warm shower and then drink some caffeine.

I'd successfully gotten through customs, collected my luggage from the conveyor belt after internally stressing that it had gotten left behind because it was one of the last suitcases to show its face, and then made my way to the train station.

I bought myself a thirteen-euro train ticket to get me into the city centre of Milan, where I'd booked to stay in a hostel for the next two nights, only to realise a few minutes later that all train trips had been cancelled for the rest of the afternoon. Brilliant.

I stood in the middle of the platform, staring at the signs above me, trying to figure out how I was now supposed to get into the city.

"Are you wanting to go to Milano Centrale?"

An American guy, who'd obviously seen me looking like a lost puppy, approached me.

"Yes, I am. How exactly are we meant to get there now?" I asked him in frustration.

"If we get a few of us together, we could split the fare for a taxi if you'd like?"

At this point, I didn't care how. I just wanted to get to my destination.

"Yep, sounds good to me!"

I sat in the back of the cab, watching the metres tick over.

"This is going to be a very expensive journey," I said to the girl sitting next to me, who'd also jumped in with us.

When we arrived at our destination about forty-five minutes later, the American guy paid the driver for the outrageously overpriced 120€ taxi ride and then waited for us to give him our share of the fare.

Shit. I don't know how I'm going to pay him. I started to worry.

"I'm so sorry. I don't have any cash on me. Can I do a bank transfer?" I asked him.

"Don't worry about it. You just got a free ride," he replied, clearly not wanting to deal with the hassle of an international transfer.

"Oh no, I feel terrible. Surely there's a way," I persisted.

"No, really, it's fine."

"Thank you so much. That's very kind of you." I grabbed my suitcase and backpack and headed towards my hostel, feeling very grateful to have finally arrived at my destination.

* * * * *

I'd booked a four-bed female dorm, and being my first-ever hostel experience, I was a little nervous about bunking with a bunch of girls I didn't know.

I checked in, paid two euros for a fresh towel and got straight into the lift to take my things up to my room.

As I opened the door to an empty dorm, I was immediately put off by how cramped the space was. There were two sets of bunk beds adjacent to one another, a block of small storage lockers for our belongings, and hardly any room for me to open up my suitcase.

It's only two nights, you'll be fine, I tried to reassure myself.

I unzipped my suitcase, picked out some clean clothes and jumped straight into the shower to freshen up.

That feels better.

I climbed up the ladder to the top bunk, flopped myself onto the thin foam mattress and took a deep breath in, thankful to finally have some peace and quiet. I decided to rest my eyes for a few minutes before venturing out to explore the city – it was only nine o'clock in the morning, and I knew I couldn't let myself fall asleep just yet.

The silence was soon disturbed when I heard people on the other side of the door trying to get in.

That didn't last long.

I quickly sat up as two of my roommates barged in.

"Hi," I said quietly and smiled at them.

"Oh, hello." They briefly looked at me, clearly not interested in engaging in any further conversation, but in all honesty, neither was I.

They fiddled about, unpacking clothes from their suitcases and walking in and out of the bathroom. I could feel myself getting more and more agitated. I knew hostels were all about meeting new people, making friends and having fun, but I honestly couldn't think of anything I felt like doing less in that moment.

After a few minutes of deliberating various options in my head, I took myself downstairs to the reception desk.

"Hi, I've just checked into a shared dorm, but I'm wondering if you have any private rooms available for the next two nights?"

The lady looked at me with a puzzled look on her face.

"I can check for you, but is everything okay? Can I help with something?"

"No, no, everything is fine. I've just changed my mind and would really like my own space." I stood there waiting patiently, desperately hoping that the universe was on my side.

"We have one left," she said, looking up at me and smiling.

"Perfect, I'll take it, please!"

I didn't even ask how much extra it was going to cost me, and at two hundred dollars per night, the price was absolutely not in my budget, but I knew the privacy was going to be worth every extra dollar.

I felt my anxiety immediately dissipate as I opened the door to my very own private space before noticing an interesting quote that caught my eye, plastered on the wall above the single bed, in beautiful large red writing, 'Tourists don't know where they've been. Travellers don't know where they're going – Paul Theroux.'

Maybe soon, I'll start to feel more like a traveller, I thought to myself.

* * * * *

I'd bought a SIM card from a Vodafone shop just outside the train station, much cheaper than any plan advertised at the airport, but annoyingly, I had been told that it could take a few hours for the roaming data to kick in. Thankfully, the receptionist back at the hostel had given me some information about where the key tourist destinations were, so I decided to put my memory to the test and follow my intuition.

I squeezed myself onto the jam-packed metro to head towards Duomo, which was the name of the stop but also the third-largest cathedral in the world.

For some reason, the train had conveniently skipped that stop, so I got off at the next one, hoping I'd be able to make my way back on foot.

Standing amongst all the other confused faces was an older Scottish couple holding their map out in front of them, trying to figure out which direction they needed to go.

"Are you, by any chance, looking for Duomo?" I asked them, hoping they might be able to help me.

"Yes, that's where we are going now. Well, trying to anyway," they laughed. "Feel free to tag along with us if you'd like."

I didn't want to cramp their style, but I was grateful for their offer as my phone was still of no use to me. With their old school paper map informed directions, we eventually found our way to Cathedral Square, and there stood a building that took nearly six centuries to finish. It was one of the most impressive, intricately designed buildings I'd ever seen.

As we stood in line, waiting to enter this monumental structure, I had the pleasure of getting to know some more about my new friends. They had two grown daughters, around the same age as me, one of who had bought them the flights to Milan for a long weekend.

We exchanged mobile numbers, and I ended up spending the next two days exploring Milan and visiting some beautiful sites alongside this lovely couple.

"You can be our adopted daughter for the weekend. And if you ever want to visit Scotland, we have a spare room for you," they kindly offered.

"Thank you so much. I'd love to visit Scotland, so I might just have to take you up on that offer one day!" They truly made my initial experience of being so far away from home a little less challenging.

"Maybe people aren't leaving you. Maybe the Universe is leaving room in your life for people who appreciate and reciprocate the love you share."

– Vex King

39

After spending the last two nights in Milan, I had finally arrived at what was going to be my new home for the next few months. My host mum, Bianca, was waiting for me out the front of the large wooden doors with a huge smile on her face. She had a very slim build, was slightly taller than me, and was wearing dark navy jeans with a lightweight jacket that covered her noticeably gorgeous olive-toned skin.

"Ciao, Ebonie! How are you?" She enthusiastically greeted me with a traditional air kiss on the left and right side of my cheeks.

"Ciao Bianca! I'm good, thank you, now that I'm here! I'm so sorry, my maps took me in the wrong direction," I admitted, relieved to have finally found her.

"How are you?"

"I'm fine, thank you. Come in," she said, motioning me inside.

I followed closely behind her as she took hold of my luggage and wheeled it towards the lift, showing me how to get to the third floor.

The moment I stepped inside their simple yet elegant two-story apartment, I was immediately welcomed by their extremely playful, medium-sized, chestnut-coloured dog, Spritz, who sprinted towards me, wiggling his entire body with excitement.

"Oh wait, it's really heavy. Are you sure you're okay with that?" I asked as Bianca proceeded to carry my twenty-five-kilogram suitcase up the wooden floored, curved staircase before I even had the chance to help her.

"Yes, don't worry. It's fine," She replied, clearly struggling to make it to the top.

She showed me through to her eldest daughter's bedroom, which was where I was going to be sleeping for the next few months while Kira was in Florida on an exchange, completing her second last year of high school. She had been there for about nine months already and was due back at the end of June.

"Wow, this room is massive!" I said to Bianca as I stood in the doorway, taking it all in. There was a comfortable-looking single bed in the back left corner, a white wooden desk up against the opposite wall, a white chest of drawers to the right and a large section of unoccupied space in the middle.

No chance of me feeling cramped in here, I thought.

Bianca put down my suitcase and then showed me where I could put my clothes.

"I must get back to work, but Anna will be walking home from school in a couple of hours. You unpack and get settled. Tell me if you need anything."

The first thing I did was remove my filthy aeroplane clothes from my backpack and put a load of washing on before completely emptying my suitcase and neatly placing everything in its new spot. My mind immediately felt a little less shambled.

* * * * *

I was sitting downstairs in the kitchen chatting to Bianca while she prepared pasta for Anna and her friend for lunch.

"Bianca, do you mind if we go through exactly what my duties are as an au pair for Anna?" Being twelve, I knew that she didn't need 'babysitting' as such or help with much at all, for that matter, but I wanted to be totally clear on what my expectations were within the household before she got home.

"Sure. Anna walks by herself to and from school every day, but she has gymnastics on Tuesday and Thursday evenings from six to seven, and I'd like you to walk with her because it gets dark. Sometimes, she might need help with her English homework, but the main thing is that she doesn't like being left at home alone. So, if I need to go out in the day, I'd need you to stay with her," Bianca explained.

"Of course! Is that all?" I replied, thinking that it all sounded very simple. "Are you sure there's nothing else I can help with?"

"No. That's all. Just spend time with her when you are both here at home."

I didn't realise I was going to have so much free time on my hands, but I certainly wasn't complaining.

Having an au pair was not exactly a new phenomenon to Anna. Right from when they had their first child seventeen years ago, Bianca and her husband, Dario, had always enjoyed having someone foreign living with them, learning about different cultures and practising different languages, particularly English. They'd had au pairs come to live with them from all over the world: South Africa, Spain, Syria, America – I was the first Australian – so the pressure was on to make a good first impression!

It was about two o'clock in the afternoon when we heard the buzzer ring. As Bianca rushed over to the front door to let the girls in, I stood up out of my chair and prepared myself to meet my host child for the first time.

Anna walked into the room and removed her bright white sneakers to put them in the shoe cupboard. It was clearly a no-shoes-in-the-house kind of thing – something I was very used to.

She turned around to see me standing in the kitchen.

"Hi!" she said joyfully with a huge grin on her face before coming over to give me a welcoming hug.

She was fairly short for her age, but I could see straight away that she was going to grow up to be a very beautiful young lady. She was wearing khaki cargo pants with a cropped t-shirt and a grey hooded jacket over the top.

Very trendy.

She had a slim build and gorgeously tanned skin, just like her mother, and her straight-cut brunette hair sat just below her shoulders.

We sat at the dining table together while they ate their lunch and told Bianca about their day, conversing through a combination of English and Italian.

Anna was fluent in English – when she spoke, she sounded like a young American girl, with hardly any hint of an Italian accent – it was impressive.

* * * * *

It was just after seven-thirty in the evening, and I was sitting on Anna's bed with my back resting up against the wall, watching her prance around her bedroom with a notepad and pen in her hand, writing down a list of movies that she wanted us to watch together over the next few months: the entire Harry Potter series, Rapunzel, Tangled, Moana, The Croods, Alvin and the Chipmunks, the list went on. If watching movies every night was considered to be one of my duties, I was absolutely living an easy life.

My stomach had started rumbling over an hour ago, and I was beginning to wonder what time dinner was going to be ready.

"What time do you usually eat dinner?" I questioned Anna as I looked down at my phone to see the time.

"It depends, but usually around eight-thirty if we eat before Dad gets home from work." I lifted my eyebrows in surprise and suddenly felt my anxiety starting to take over my thoughts.

Another hour!

"Why, what time do you usually eat?" she asked.

"Normally around six-thirty, so eating later is going to take some getting used to," I laughed, trying to hide any sign of distress I was feeling.

It's a running joke amongst most of my friends at home that I am a grandma. I am a sucker for a routine. I'd have my dinner ready and eaten before six-thirty, be in bed by eight-thirty, and be asleep by nine, with an alarm set for five o'clock to go to the gym before starting work.

But when I arrived in Italy, I knew that the grandma in me would have to take a back seat and learn to adjust to a completely different lifestyle – a much later lifestyle.

The thought of having to wait to eat dinner until after eight-thirty in the evening was something I knew I would struggle with most, but I could never put my finger on exactly why… was it because I was anxious about being so hungry that maybe I'd end up overeating? Or was it because I simply didn't have the control to choose when I could eat?

I'd often try my best to find out what was on the menu for dinner each evening, mostly so that I could plan the rest of my daily intake around that specific meal.

I'd start by asking Bianca if Dario would be home for dinner – some nights, he would stay in Milan for work; otherwise, he would usually be home after nine o'clock in the evening – or I'd ask if she needed any help preparing the meal, which would usually prompt her to tell me what she had planned.

Bianca was very health conscious and took pride in what she put into her body, something that I found very reassuring. She went to the fruit and vegetable market every Friday afternoon and would come home with two full bags of fresh produce and about ten different varieties of green leafy vegetables, some that I didn't even know existed.

She didn't cook a lot of meat for the family, but when she did, it was high quality and ethically sourced from their local butcher. Although she loved her typical Italian dishes, most of what she cooked for us was not of Italian cuisine. Some of her staple meals included vegetable soup, grilled fish, lentils and other legumes, chicken and salad piadina, and vegetable couscous. We also always had an abundance of organic sourdough that she would buy for thirteen euros a loaf! Price was never a concern for Bianca – her health was always more important. It was uncanny just how much she reminded me of my mum.

"Mum wants to know what pizza you want," Anna said to me as she walked back into her room and came to sit on the chair beside me to continue doing her English homework.

"Oh, is that what we're having tonight?" For an Italian family, we actually didn't get pizza very often, but every time we did, I knew that it would awaken the anxiety lying dormant inside of me once again. It wasn't that I didn't want the delicately blistered wood-fired pizza because I did; a little part of me even got excited at the thought of devouring an entire pizza. But that's where the excitement abruptly stopped, at an idea, because I didn't want to allow myself to eat the whole thing.

"What's the place called?" I asked. Anna gave me the name of the restaurant, and I studied the online menu intently, trying to find the healthiest, lowest-calorie-looking pizza.

We sat at the dinner table, each of us with our full-sized pizza in front of us, using a knife to cut it into slices because, apparently, the restaurants don't do that for you in Italy. I watched as Anna absolutely demolished the entire thing as if she'd never been fed before, Bianca and Dario not far behind her.

Once I'd eaten the centre of my pizza and all the toppings, with a hint of guilt hiding behind every mouthful, I couldn't stop myself from picking at the thicker bits of crust that I'd pushed to the side until I had pretty much devoured the entire thing. This was when the unwelcoming tsunami of guilty thoughts flooded my mind.

I can't believe I just ate the whole pizza. Now I've overeaten, who knows how many calories I just had. I should have stopped myself.

When we were dismissed from the table, Anna and I went upstairs to watch a movie together, while I continued to fight against my anxiety to calm the storm that was threatening to erupt inside of my head.

I'm proud of myself for eating the whole thing, I thought. I really enjoyed it, every bite tasted so good, and I'm actually satisfied.

There was a time when the anxiety would be too overwhelming, too powerful and robust for the more rational thoughts to squeeze their way through to the front of my mind, and I would just crumble in a heap.

Step by step, I was getting stronger, more resilient and able to win the battle that, once upon a time, had always beaten me.

*"The journey changes you; it should change you.
It leaves marks on your memory, on your consciousness,
on your heart and on your body. You take something
with you, and hopefully, you leave something
good behind too."*

– Anthony Bourdain

40

It was the beginning of June when Aunty Jan came to visit me for a week in Turin after spending the last four weeks travelling through the south of France. It had only been about three weeks since I'd last seen her, after spending a magical weekend together, exploring the city of Nice and admiring the fact that people either walked or drove the most luxurious brands of cars through the streets of Monte Carlo. It was said to be one of the richest cities in the world and I was happy to have ticked that one off the bucket list because it was safe to say I was absolutely out of my league.

We had met for an evening meal at one of my favourite traditional Italian restaurants down the road from where my host family lived. The waitress guided us towards the outdoor dining area to our elegantly prepared table and then gave us some time to view the menu. When the waitress came back to take our order, I decided that I wanted to try the beef agnolotti pasta and Aunty Jan chose a classic vegetarian pizza. She then proceeded to lay the white linen napkins across our laps, and we waited patiently for our meal to arrive.

In the midst of our conversation, I began to express to Aunty Jan how much I'd felt I had grown over the last three months of living abroad, how well I had coped with such a significant change to my lifestyle and how proud I was with how quickly and easily I had adapted. It was something I never thought I'd be able to do, and I had successfully proven myself wrong.

Aunty Jan looked at me, her eyes shining sincerely.

"I know your mum would be incredibly proud of you, Eb, as we all are."

A smile tugged at the corners of my mouth, and I felt my energy suddenly lift.

"Thank you; all I ever wanted was to make her proud," I said. I looked down at my half-eaten bowl of agnolotti and then stuck my fork into another piece of beef-filled pasta.

"Can I ask you something?"

"Yes, of course. Anything," she replied.

"I've always wondered… what were your immediate thoughts when I phoned you that day to tell you that Mum had died?" It was a question I had always wanted to ask, but it just never felt like the right moment.

Aunty Jan put down her knife and fork and wiped her mouth with her white linen napkin while taking a moment to ponder my rather significant question before answering.

"Well, of course, I was in shock. I struggled to comprehend it at first, but I knew I had to remain strong for you. I remember telling you that what your mum had done was a tragedy, but her pain and suffering had gotten all too much for her to cope with, and she couldn't push through any longer."

Her brows furrowed, and the corners of her lips drew down as she continued to cast her mind back to the very moment her life also changed forever.

"I remember feeling extremely let down by your mum. I always used to call myself her 'prop.' We would talk for hours, and I'd try to help her in any way I could. I suggested volunteer work, professional help, anything really, that would get her out of the house. And when it would come time for me to leave, I'd feel a sense of hope, confident that together, we had taken a healthy step forward. But it was like the moment I walked out that front door, her demons overpowered any positive influence I thought I had. She was already heading in the opposite direction," she sighed heavily.

"Do you know when it all started? What made her so mentally unwell?" I asked yet another deep and heavy question, but I couldn't help myself. Aunty Jan knew Mum better than anyone; she was the closest I was going to get to Mum answering these questions herself.

"I remember how incredibly happy she was when you were a young child; you were the light of her entire world, and you gave her so much purpose. She put a significant amount of time and energy into your learning. You read books together, sang nursery rhymes, danced to the Wiggles, helped her bake her favourite banana cake." I smiled as some of these memories suddenly came flooding back into my mind.

"She went back to teaching when you were about two or three and seemed to manage quite well. Like any marriage, your parents had their ups and downs, nothing they couldn't overcome, but always lingering in the back of her mind was this deep concern about providing a loving family unit for you; she was always so anxious about failing you in some way, and not being able to give you all the things a happy family could bring." She stopped for a second.

"I truly believe that it was the overwhelming pressure she put on herself to be the best in every aspect of her life that made her become so sick – physically and mentally."

I nodded in complete agreement.

"Then she came down with a terrible bout of glandular fever, which meant she had to take a significant amount of time off work. It was soon after this that she moved into the spare room. I remember this being a very confusing time for you."

"Oh yes, I didn't know when that started. I don't even remember them ever sleeping together," I replied.

"I think she hoped it would ease some of the tension between her and your dad while she was unwell. It took months for her to recover from the virus, which obviously put more strain on their financial situation. This was also when all her ongoing health issues began – the constant stomach issues, body rashes and chronic fatigue. She started to see the naturopath because she became very sensitive to any medication or drug that wasn't natural. Your dad tried to do everything he could to help, but it certainly took a toll on their relationship, and he started to become very frustrated. He was working even harder to make up for the money that your mum wasn't bringing in, but I know he always felt that she could have done more. This was the catalyst to their separation."

"I honestly don't blame him for leaving. Even after they'd broken up and she was constantly complaining about being sick, having stomach cramps or not wanting to get out of bed, I always felt that she wasn't trying hard enough to get better. It was like she just couldn't be bothered with life anymore."

My mum lived like a recluse. She would force herself to go to work just so she could make ends meet for us, but by the time Friday rolled around, she would be totally exhausted; she wouldn't want to go anywhere or do anything. The weekends were a time for her to rest and recover, to prepare herself to get through the next week. I wasn't allowed to have friends over because it would make her too anxious, and apart from saying hello to the neighbours on rare occasions, Aunty Jan was basically the only visitor she had.

"I felt a sense of relief when she started taking you to church on a Sunday evening," Aunty Jan continued.

"I was hopeful that this was exactly what she needed in her life – a group of beautiful people that she would feel comfortable around and confide in if she needed. But I was disappointed when I heard her say, 'None of them want to listen to me; they all have enough of their own problems.' She just couldn't see the benefit in being open with other people."

It made me sad that my mum never got the help that she needed. She had always sent me to see a counsellor or a psychologist but never got the professional help she needed for herself, and I know that it was this lack of sharing her thoughts and fears with others that dug her deeper into this dark hole of depression that no one seemed to be able to pull her out of.

I looked at Aunty Jan and took a deep breath in.

"I think she planned out the whole thing. I think she knew she was going to end her life and how she was going to do it; it was just a matter of when," I said.

"I remember the week before it all happened, I flew down to Melbourne to visit my family, and Mum was supposed to come with me, but at the last minute, she rang my uncle, explaining she would send me on my own because she had some things to sort out."

I couldn't know for sure, but I had this intuitive feeling that my mum had spent that time putting as much as she could in place for me so she knew that I'd be okay when she was no longer around.

"Yes, I think you're right," Aunty Jan's tone lowered. "But I know that we did everything we could to help her, and at the end of the day, it was her choice. No one was going to stop her."

"I don't think I'll ever be able to thank you enough for everything you and Rex have done for me in my life. I wouldn't be the person I am today without you, and I hope you know how incredibly grateful I am."

Aunty Jan's eyes began to well as she listened to the gratitude I was trying to express. For the last twelve years, she had been my safety net, the person I knew I could rely on the most, my biggest support, and my heart needed her to know how lucky I felt to have had her by my side all of this time. I could never put into words how much it meant to me.

"When it feels scary to jump, that's exactly when you jump, otherwise you end up staying in the same place your whole life."

– Abel Morales

41

I'd been living with my Italian host family for just over five months, thoroughly enjoying being able to fully embrace the Italian culture and live like an Italian local. I couldn't believe how quickly time had flown by. Although I had successfully continued to maintain my daily Duolingo streak, I had also decided that it would be a good idea to hire a private tutor and actually try to learn the language properly, which helped a lot. I had reached the point where I could listen, understand and read Italian a whole lot better than I could speak it, but it was my lack of confidence that needed the most attention.

It was the beginning of August, and summer was in full swing, with days of extreme humidity and temperatures reaching a high of forty degrees across most parts of Italy. My host mum had previously warned me that Turin would become much like a ghost town during the summer vacation, as families fled the city to stay in their holiday homes by the seaside or in the mountains. She wasn't wrong.

The air was still, and the sun's rays radiated off the tall, old concrete buildings as I walked through the streets of Turin. The sweat began to drip from my skin the moment I stepped outside. It was almost unbearable.

Thankfully, it wasn't long until I got to see a familiar face again. Maddie was set to be flying from the land down under to meet me in Istanbul at the end of the month before we began our five-week adventure together, kicking off with an iconic nine-day guided tour through parts of Turkey and a three-day cruise around the Greek Islands. We had then planned to travel across to the south of Italy to visit Sorrento, Isle of Capri and Pompeii before venturing up to Venice, across to Barcelona and finishing in the vibrant city of London.

My original plan was to then fly home at the end of this wild Italian ride and return to my old Australian life, but I wasn't quite ready for this journey to end just yet. I still had so much more of the world that I wanted to see, so many more adventures to encounter, and so much more growth to achieve. I just had to figure out where my next move was going to be.

Honestly, the thought of being back in an English-speaking country was extremely inviting, so I decided to apply for another working holiday visa, but this time, for the UK. Suddenly, the anxiety of trying to find a place to live and a job to pay my bills had come to visit me once again. I had no idea what my life in the UK looked like – I planned to rock up in London and hope that I would figure it all out within a week of my arrival, but honestly, having nothing set in stone terrified me. I kept telling myself it was all going to work out, that it would all fall into place exactly how it was supposed to. I chose to trust the process.

Prior to leaving Australia, I had reached out to a few neurological rehabilitation centres across parts of Europe that were very similar to Making Strides, two of which I received a positive response from and were more than happy to have me come to visit their clinics for a day while I was in the area.

When I realised that I was actually going to be living in the UK for the foreseeable future, I decided to stick my feelers out once again, but this time, to enquire about a potential career opportunity at one of the neurological centres not far out of London. Being able to use my degree was certainly more appealing to me than working in some monotonous hospitality job.

* * * * *

We thought we better make ourselves comfortable, knowing that we were going to be sitting on this tour bus for the next three hours while we made our way to Pamukkale, a popular tourist destination in southwest Turkey. Pamukkale is known for its stunning landscape of white travertine terraces and mineral-rich thermal pools believed to have healing properties.

I looked down at my phone to check the notification that had just come through. It was the company I had enquired about just outside of London. I opened the email, and a bubble of joy expanded in my chest. They were, in fact, actively hiring!

"Look!" I turned towards Maddie grinning from ear to ear, shoving the phone in her face. "They've offered me an interview!"

"See! I knew they would," she replied.

I followed through with the interview process, and two days later, I received the confirmation. I had successfully landed a position as an exercise physiologist and secured a place to live just around the corner. I couldn't believe how easily it had all fallen into place. Two weeks prior to arriving in London, I knew exactly what my plan was, and I couldn't have been happier.

"Are you healed or just isolated with no one to trigger you?"

– Steven Bartlett

42

I was incredibly excited to be boarding my very first cruise ship around the Greek Islands. It was two-hundred and fifteen metres long, twenty-eight metres wide, and had a total of ten decks, an outdoor swimming pool, a gym, a spa and multiple bars. Our three-night package included a buffet for breakfast, lunch and dinner, with the option to enjoy an à la carte menu in the evening, as well as complimentary beer, wine, spirits, soft drinks and a selection of cocktails that were under seven euros – Maddie absolutely wouldn't let those go to waste.

I stood in the queue behind Maddie, eagerly waiting to be seated for our very first buffet breakfast the following morning, and I caught myself thinking, how can the one thing that excites me so much be the very thing that causes me the most anxiety?

I could see from a short distance all the food that was on offer, and I couldn't wait to load up my plate, but at the same time, I was so paranoid about letting my hunger take control and being unable to stop myself from eating too much.

My thoughts were disrupted when we reached the front of the line.

"How many people?" the lady asked.

"Just two, please," I answered.

A waiter came over to collect us and motioned us towards our table.

"Please follow me."

I hung my bag over the back of my chair and made my way towards the food station. I grabbed a plate and waited as the line of people slowly moved past the selection of bread, cereals, fruits and yogurts and towards the hot breakfast dishes. There was so much choice I was struggling to decide what to put on my plate. I wanted it all, but I also didn't want to give in to my temptations.

When I sat down at my seat, I immediately wanted to know how many calories I had put on my plate. As I pierced my knife into the perfectly cooked poached egg and watched the bright orange yolk run onto the piece of toast below it, I started to mentally calculate the calories in the foods I knew off the top of my head: two eggs, seventy calories each, a piece of wholemeal bread, about one hundred calories. A tub of plain low-fat yogurt, the label conveniently told me it had eighty calories. A bowl of mixed fruit, let's say one hundred calories. About four hundred and twenty calories so far. My anxiety settled.

I'll go back for seconds, but just load up on the stir-fried vegetables. Then I'll let myself pick one dessert and go to the gym when we get back from our tour, I told myself.

I stood in front of the dessert table admiring the sweet treats, trying to decide which one I wanted most, even though my belly felt like it was going to explode.

"I'll take a chocolate muffin back to our room and save it for later," I told Maddie as I picked one up and wrapped it in a napkin to help disguise it on our way out.

We had just arrived at the docking station in Athens and were sitting in the common area, waiting with three thousand other people to be called off the ship to take part in our first tour of the Acropolis. The organised tours were being called first, so it was going to take at least another thirty minutes before it was our turn to disembark.

"I'm just going to go back to the room to use the toilet. I won't be long," I told Maddie as I stood up from the lounge chair and grabbed the key out of my bag before handing her the rest of my belongings to look after.

When I opened the door to our room, my eyes were drawn to the muffin sitting on the table, and the temptation to eat it was almost irresistible. I stared at it for a few seconds.

There are probably about two hundred calories in this thing—calories I don't need and calories I should save for later. I'll just have one bite.

One bite turned into me standing over the empty toilet bowl in our small cabin bathroom, with more than half of the chocolate muffin shoved in my mouth at once.

Why am I doing this again? I thought.

It tasted so good I just wanted more. I proceeded to finish the rest of the muffin but didn't allow myself to swallow any of it. In the moment, it felt good. I was able to taste the deliciousness without the guilt. But afterwards, I just felt disappointed in myself.

Five weeks of travelling was the longest I'd ever been out of a routine. I was eating lots of different foods and unable to have a consistent exercise regime. Luckily, we were doing a lot of walking every day along our travels, which helped to ease my anxiety a little, but it didn't stop me from thinking about every calorie I consumed. The anxious thoughts were definitely not as loud as they had been in the past, and I felt more in control, but they were still there, and it made me wonder if they would ever fully disappear.

"It's not something you get over;
it's just something you get through."

– Willie Nelson

43

It was the day that held - and still holds - a very significant place in my heart – the anniversary of my mum's death. A day that I always took a few moments to sit quietly, reflect and allow myself to feel whatever emotions came up for me at that time. My usual tradition was to light a candle, play my mum's favourite song and write to her in my journal. However, circumstances were a little different this year. Maddie and I were in the midst of our travels and had just set off on our next road trip down to Bath in England. It was a beautiful day, very fresh, but the sun was shining, and there was not a cloud in the sky.

I turned to look at Maddie as she was focused intently on the road ahead of us.

"It's mum's anniversary today," I said.

"I know. I thought about that this morning and wanted to say something. How are you feeling?"

"I'm fine. But I'd like to play her song if that's okay?"

Amazing Grace by a female acapella group, who sing the most beautiful version of this song, is the track I play every year. I got it up on my phone and pressed play. I rested my head back on the headrest and looked out the window as it started to play through the speakers of the car.

'My chains are gone; I've been set free. My god, my Saviour has ransomed me. And like a flood, His mercy reigns. Unending love, amazing grace.'

My favourite verse, which resonates so perfectly.

I closed my eyes as a solemn tear fell down my cheek.

"I love you," I whispered.

* * * * *

Our time spent travelling around Europe had come to an end, and it felt like I was saying goodbye to my significant other. Maddie and I had been by each other's side, seven days a week, twenty-four hours a day, for a total of five weeks and once again, I wasn't ready to say goodbye.

Our final hour together was spent on the train to Heathrow Airport so I could help her check in her bag before we went our separate ways.

"I don't want you to go," I whispered as I wrapped my arms around her shoulders and squeezed her tight.

"Trust me, I'd much rather be staying here with you," she said. She could tell I was trying my best to hold back my tears.

"Please don't cry. You're going to make me cry, and then I won't be able to stop. I have to look somewhat presentable when I walk into the Qantas lounge," she laughed. She got out her pack of tissues and handed me one.

"I'm going to miss you so much. Have a safe flight home, and call me when you land at your stopover. I love you," I quickly turned around and began walking in the opposite direction to stop myself from getting too emotional. I looked back over my shoulder to wave one final goodbye. As soon as she was out of my sight, the ugly crying commenced.

In typical UK style, it was raining that evening and without realising, the bus to take me to my new home wasn't leaving for another ninety minutes.

Great.

I decided to catch a rather expensive Uber – I couldn't be bothered with the hassle. It was worth every penny, knowing that I wouldn't have to sit and wait and then walk thirty minutes from the bus stop to my house in the pouring rain.

* * * * *

It was my first night in my new place, and I knew my housemate was away for the weekend visiting his family. Maddie and I had already dropped off my bags, made my bed and done a big food shop a few days prior to her departure, so it was all set up for me when I arrived.

I had been so excited all day to finally be able to settle in and sleep in what I could now call my bed, but as I walked through the front door to a very quiet and empty apartment, a dark cloud of fear began to loom over me.

This feels very strange, I thought.

I decided I needed to distract myself from the unwanted feelings that were starting to erupt inside of me. It felt like my body was shaking from the inside out, and I didn't know how to control it.

I started to unpack my bags, organise my cupboards and drawers, put a load of washing on and then realised how late it was getting.

Not even three hours had passed since I'd said goodbye to Maddie at the airport, but I needed to hear her voice once more before she would be unreachable for the next seven hours.

"Hello gorgeous, how are you settling in tonight?" she answered.

"Not good. I don't like this feeling; I miss you so much already."

The cloud that was hovering above me suddenly decided to let go and the tears began to spill over the sides of my eyes, streaming down my cheeks. The deep, heavy pit I had in my stomach made me feel like I was going to be sick. I didn't know what to do to make myself feel any better. I just wanted Maddie to be right here with me.

"Oh, baby girl, please don't be upset. You're only feeling this way because you're not used to me not being there. It will get easier, I promise. It's just going to take some time to adjust," she said, trying to reassure me.

"But what if I can't do it? What if I've made the wrong decision, and I need to come home?" I felt a paralysing anxiety begin to take over.

"Then you just come home," she replied bluntly. "But I know that won't happen."

I guess it was just as simple as that. If I really didn't like it, if things didn't turn out how I'd hoped, nothing was stopping me from jumping on a plane home.

* * * * *

I woke up the following morning, walked over to my bedroom window to open the curtains, and, to my surprise, the sun was shining.

At least, this is a positive start to my day, I thought.

My body continued to tremble at the thought of being so alone. I felt sick, I had no appetite, and all I wanted to do was crawl back into bed and hibernate. I didn't. At least not in that moment.

I forced myself to eat breakfast and called one of my best friends from home, hoping this would ease the knot in my stomach. It didn't. The heaviness in my chest was becoming so unbearable it felt like nothing I did was helping. I walked into my room and closed the door behind me, even though no one else was home. I pulled back the covers on my neatly made bed and curled up in a tight ball, hugging the pillow next to me, hoping it would provide me with some form of comfort. I let it all out and cried until I couldn't anymore.

* * * * *

Getting through the first week was tough. I was in a completely new environment, with no one to meet up with or talk to, and I had no idea what to do with my time.

Two weeks went by, and I successfully made it through my first full week of work. It felt so good to be back in a somewhat familiar environment, doing something I knew I was good at and feeling like I was helping to make a difference in people's lives once again. My colleagues were so welcoming, and I was enjoying getting to know everyone, excited about hopefully being able to form some genuine friendships along the way. Things were definitely starting to look up and I knew I had made the right decision.

"All of it is life. All of it is precious. Don't waste any of it doing something you don't want to do. And do all of it with the people you love."

– Sir Richard Branson

44

It was the middle of winter, and the coats were out in full force in most parts of the northern hemisphere. Escaping to a somewhat warmer climate where the sun actually made an appearance seemed extremely appealing so I decided to book a rather spontaneous three-night getaway to Morocco to meet up with one of my dear friends from Australia, Jackson. Jackson had been staying in Lisbon for the previous five weeks and was doing some last-minute travel before heading back home.

The moment I stepped off the plane at Marrakech airport, I realised how pleasant it was not to be struck with a sudden gust of wind that pierced straight through my body – it was the warm change in temperature I was hoping for.

I hurried through customs and walked out the front doors, frantically looking left and right, and beamed with excitement when I spotted his familiar face.

There he was, waiting behind the rails, greeting me with an electronic sign on his phone that read 'EBS.' I immediately ran towards him with my arms outstretched in front of me, squealing with happiness, before gently colliding into him with a warm embrace.

"Oh my goodness, it's so good to see you! I missed you so much!" I exclaimed as we continued to hold the moment for as long as possible.

"How was your flight? How was Lisbon? Ah, there's so much to catch up on!" I started rambling, not knowing where to even begin.

Our taxi dropped us at an unfamiliar location and handed us to a couple of young guys who had clearly been asked to lead us towards our hotel. The roaming data on our phones still hadn't kicked in, so we had no way of confirming we were heading in the right direction.

Jackson and I continued to tentatively follow them through the dark, smelly and chaotic back streets of Marrakech. Scooters and motorbikes flew past us with no sense of direction and I looked back at Jackson, who was walking closely behind me. I had concern written all over my face – it really didn't feel like we were heading towards the hotel we had booked, according to the photos we had seen online.

"Excuse me, do you mind if we look at the maps on your phone, please?" Jackson asked politely, stopping the boys in their tracks.

"It's okay, it's okay. We take you to your hotel. It is this way," they beckoned, trying to reassure us.

"Can we please look at your phone first?" Jackson persisted.

After a few minutes of scrambling to find the correct address, we were relieved to discover these two strangers were, in fact, taking us to the proper location.

After a somewhat sketchy start to our evening, we finally arrived at our hotel – a Riad, known as a traditional Moroccan palace with an indoor garden and courtyard. The address was correct, but the outside had us seriously questioning our decision. It looked like we'd just arrived at some spooky dungeon with scaffolding surrounding the outskirts of the building. We were enthusiastically greeted by the receptionist, Aiyub, who welcomed us inside and then proceeded to explain to us that we would not be staying at this particular Riad because the shower in our room was broken.

Perfect, I thought to myself.

I dropped my heavy backpack to the floor, looked up at Jackson and started to laugh at how incredibly well our night was going so far.

Before moving to the sister Riad, we were first directed to the dining area upstairs to be seated for our evening meal, which, thankfully, we had pre-booked prior to our arrival. It was about nine o'clock by this point, and I was starving.

We kicked off our three-course dinner with an entrée of Moroccan bread and a large bowl of salad, followed by a main meal that was served in a traditional ceramic tajine cooking vessel. My eyes lit up with excitement as Aiyub removed the lid, revealing what was underneath – a very large serving of authentic Moroccan couscous topped with slow-cooked chicken and assorted stewed vegetables. One spoonful after another, the exotic flavours continued to explode in my mouth. It was delicious. For dessert, the online menu read assorted Moroccan pastries, but instead, we were presented with a bowl of whole fruits: apples, mandarins and bananas – one for each of us.

"Can't say I've ever been served a fruit bowl for dessert before," I joked. I was so full that I didn't feel like eating dessert anyway.

A few minutes later, Aiyub walked out of the kitchen with a huge smile on his face, holding a plate of six assorted cookies with a layer of icing as thick as the biscuit beneath it. He placed them down on the table in front of us.

"Now, you won't find these anywhere else in the world!" he said.

"Oh, I'm sure of that," Jackson laughed. It was quite comical, really.

I gave Jackson the honours of first choice. He picked the prettiest-looking cookie and took a bite.

"Ah, it tastes as stale as candle wax," he said.

I burst into laughter, slightly disappointed but not surprised by his reaction. I then reluctantly took a bite of one of them to assess them for myself.

"Yep, you're not wrong about that," I laughed.

* * * * *

The next morning we were picked up from our hotel, along with two young guys from Copenhagen and a young couple from the south of Spain. We were off on a trekking tour through the High Atlas Mountains of Morocco. It took roughly an hour and a half to drive to our starting location, which allowed us to pass through the neighbouring villages along the valley and admire the incredible landscapes that surrounded us.

When we arrived at the Berber village of Imlil, I stepped out of the van and noticed how much cooler it was than the city of Marrakech, which was going to reach a high of twenty-eight degrees. With an ascent that took us to about fifteen hundred metres above sea level, it meant we were sitting at a temperature of roughly sixteen degrees – perfect hiking temperature.

We made our way into a small room and sat ourselves down on the wooden benches, where we were introduced to our tour guide, who would be with us for the next two days. Hassan was in his late twenties, born and raised in a very small and quaint mountain settlement tucked away amongst the beautiful serenity of Toubkal Valley. He was of average height with a very slender build and spoke with a very soft and delicate voice.

"I know I might look very weak to you, but I can assure you I am not. I hike these mountains almost every day. It is my life."

Hassan went on to explain that he willingly hiked to the top of Toubkal Mountain, the highest peak in North Africa, with various tour groups, sometimes ten to fifteen times a month. It took about two to three days to reach the summit, at an elevation of 4,167 metres, and could be very dangerous during the winter months, with extremely strong winds and temperatures dropping as low as negative fifteen degrees. I knew we were in very safe hands. Our little trek was nothing compared to that, but I was incredibly excited.

* * * * *

After the first two hours of walking a solid uphill trail, we reached the highest peak of our trek, standing at roughly 2,200 metres above sea level. My jumper was off, the back of my shirt was damp from sweat, and I was grateful I wasn't doing this tour during the middle of summer. I stood at the top and looked out towards the pristine mountains that surrounded us; the air was fresh, and there was not a cloud in the sky. It was truly magical.

We walked over to where lunch was being served and sat ourselves down on the benches on either side of the small wooden table and took in the tranquil valley below us. We were promptly greeted with a large pot of mint tea, a very important part of the Moroccan culture – traditionally practised as a gesture of hospitality. The higher the tea is poured, creating more bubbles on the surface, the more welcomed the guests are. We each had a turn of pouring the tea into a glass as high as we could without spilling it over the edges.

"Higher, higher, higher," we joked with each other.

Hassan then brought out the plates and cutlery for us, and with what came out next, I knew we would not be left hungry. Our cook prepared a basket of Moroccan bread, a large plate of mixed salad with some sort of fish in the middle, a bowl of plain pasta and a traditional shakshouka, which I later found out is a North African dish of scrambled eggs in a sauce of tomatoes, onions, peppers and Moroccan spices – chef's kiss!

* * * * *

It was about three o'clock in the afternoon and time to begin the second half of our journey for the day towards the Tizi Oussem village, where we would be spending the night as a group.

Jackson and I continued to sing and dance our way down the valley, through Juniper Forest, while taking a million and one happy snaps of each other doing the most random things – pistol squatting on any aesthetically pleasing rock soon became our signature move.

Upon arrival to the Berber village, home to roughly six-hundred people, we were eagerly welcomed by about a dozen of the local young boys and girls, who wanted us to join them in playing football.

After carrying my backpack all day, I was very keen to finally put it down. I swiftly swung it off my shoulder and dropped it onto the ground before grabbing out my bottle to enjoy the last sip of water I had left. I then noticed a little boy walking over towards me. He stood next to my bag, leaning up against the wall, and looked up at me with his big beady brown eyes.

"Hello! How are you?" I asked, knowing full well he probably had no idea what I was saying. I received no response, but instead, he continued to smile nervously at me. I held out my hand next to his, and he accepted my offer, gripping it tightly. We walked down to where the other children and the rest of my group were playing together and watched them kick the ball to one another.

"Jackson, when you get the ball next, can you try to kick it over this way?"

He nodded at me, suggesting he knew exactly what I was trying to do.

When the ball came my way, I stopped it with my foot and guided it towards my little friend.

"Go on, your turn!" I encouraged him. Still holding onto my hand, he then proceeded to kick the ball with all his might and then giggled softly to himself. He looked up at me and smiled, grateful that I had given him a chance. My heart was so full.

* * * * *

As we walked into the guest house, we were all pleasantly surprised by the standard of our rooms, in comparison to the incredibly simple houses we had seen along the way, built from clay bricks and bamboo sticks, covered in red mud and dried by the sun. I'd never seen anything like it.

We had been given three separate bedrooms, with a single bed for each of us, a pillow the size of a log, and a fully equipped bathroom with a shower and hot running water. We were even given a wifi password! (Not that it worked very well). Nonetheless, this was a luxury compared to the expectation we had of sleeping on the floor with sleeping bags and using a bucket of water to bathe ourselves in. Part of me wanted to experience the full authenticity of how the Berber locals lived, to fully embrace the simple, nomadic, technology-free lifestyle that they do, but after five hours and twelve kilometres of hiking, I was very grateful to have a bed.

* * * * *

It was ten o'clock in the morning, the air was brisk, and our bellies were full from a simple but wholesome breakfast. We were ready for the next part of our adventure: four hours of hiking before taking a break for lunch and then returning to Marrakech.

As we made our way across the rugged terrain of one of Morocco's finest Atlas Mountains towards another Berber village below us, we took a moment to pause and admire the breathtaking views surrounding us.

With not a cloud in the sky and the sun's rays beaming down on my bare skin that was a little paler than normal, I felt a cool breeze gently brush over me, helping to lower my slightly raised body temperature.

I stood and watched from afar as the children ran around on the orange, dusty land beneath their dirty, worn-out shoes, laughing and screaming as they chased after their half-deflated football – not a care in the world.

"That's a nice-looking house with the blue, yellow and green painted walls," one of the guys in our group said, pointing to a small building that sat towards the top of the village.

"That's the primary school," Hassan corrected him. A building that looked like it could fit no more than a single classroom of students in it was actually the entire school. I was shocked.

I continued to observe the life of the locals before me, a life that was a complete juxtaposition to my own, and I was reminded of how truly privileged I was to live the life that I do, to have the opportunity to experience the many blessings that this world has to offer and be able to achieve them so easily, with very few restrictions.

We had covered just over five kilometres so far, and I noticed how the track was starting to get narrower, with the drop to our right becoming more precipitous as we continued to pass through the neighbouring valleys. My eyes remained glued to my feet, concentrating intently on every step as I tried to avoid the rocks that looked like they would easily dislodge. I reminded myself to look up every few minutes to soak in the feeling of serenity that encapsulated us. The views were truly remarkable.

* * * * *

Jackson laughed to himself as he gently nudged my shoulder towards the cliff face beside me, causing me to lose balance for a brief moment.

"How have you been Eb's? Really?" he asked sincerely.

I looked up at the path ahead of us and let out a little chuckle as I thought about how to answer this.

"I feel like I'm actually in a really good space at the moment," I said, deciding to begin with the positives.

"I really struggled at first. I honestly had thoughts about giving up and flying home. But now, I feel like I've really started to settle into my new routine; my place is super comfortable, I love my new job, I've met some wonderful people, and I love being able to jump across to different countries on the weekend when I feel like it."

Jackson nodded in agreement. "Yeah, that's what I've really enjoyed about being on this side of the world for the last five weeks. It's just so easy!"

"Absolutely! But, if I had a dollar for every time someone asked me why I moved from Australia to England, I'd be bloody rich," I joked.

"I do miss the Aussie sun every once and a while," I laughed again. "But the cooler weather is a nice change. I'm just choosing to embrace it all."

I took in a deep breath and decided to open up to Jackson a little more.

"I still struggle with my eating, though; the anxiety I get around food is still there. It's so much better than what it was. I know how to manage it now, and I'm proud of how much progress I've made, but sometimes I wonder if it will ever truly go away, if I'll ever be 'cured' by this little voice in the back of my head that seems to want to control my thoughts every time I eat something that I consider to be 'unhealthy.'" I said, using two fingers from each hand to gesture quotation marks.

"Before I left Oz, just after my last big olympic lifting competition, I wasn't feeling so confident in how I looked. I was just feeling a little too... bulky."

Jackson listened intently to me ramble on, so I continued.

"When I got to Italy, I was doing so much walking, over ten thousand steps most days... I also joined a gym but obviously wasn't training at the same intensity as I was used to – it was a nice change, though, and then I noticed that I was starting to lose some weight, mostly all of my muscle," I chuckled.

"Oh my goodness, I'm so weak now!" I said in a half-joking, half-serious tone.

"No, you're not. Don't be ridiculous. You still managed to pull off a pistol squat on the edge of a cliff." Jackson flippantly nudged into the side of me again.

"Yeah, but so did you! And there's absolutely no chance of me squatting one hundred kilos anymore!" I said.

"But it's obviously not my priority right now, so losing a bit of strength actually doesn't bother me, and to be honest, I feel more confident in my body than I have in a while. I just need to make sure I don't get obsessive again and keep losing weight…"

"Eb, you still look so strong. You don't need to worry about how you look," Jackson said, trying to reassure me.

"Thank you," I said timidly, trying to accept the compliment. "Anyway, apart from that, I'm really happy at the moment." I looked over at Jackson with a wide grin.

He looked up ahead of us, his head tilted slightly and his eyes narrowed. I could see his mind ticking over as if he had something else he wanted to say.

"Okay, well, here's another one for you… When has Ebs felt the most Ebs?" he said.

It was a question that no one had ever asked me before and one that I didn't really know how to answer. My mind tried to recall a recent moment in my life when I felt the most alive, a time when I felt completely content and at ease.

"Jeez, we're really diving in deep and getting sentimental today, aren't we?" I teased.

As I pondered this intriguing question a little longer, I thought maybe I didn't feel the most 'me' when I was at my happiest. What if it was actually the contrary? A time in my life when I was at my lowest and acutely aware of every physiological, emotional and psychological sensation in my body; when I was forced to turn inward, come home and decide how exactly I wanted to move forward. Maybe it was in these moments I felt the most Ebs. One foot in front of the other. And finally, that was okay.

"You can have more than one home. You can carry your roots with you and decide where they grow."

– Henning Mankell

EPILOGUE

It's been over twelve months since I left the only place I knew as home and embarked on one of the most magnificent adventures of my life. In that time, I have lived in two different regions, and visited fourteen countries, twenty-four cities and nine different islands. I have stayed in my first hostel, conquered my first driving experience on the other side of the road, and earned some extra dollars doing some English tutoring while looking after children. I have dog sat, house sat, started a new job, bought a cheap runaround car, had my first winter Christmas, significantly improved my geographical knowledge, and met some incredible people along the way. But most importantly, I have developed into a wiser, more resilient and confident person, in ways I never would have achieved if it weren't for the highs and lows of the wild rollercoaster of travel.

Nothing could have prepared me for the level of uncertainty and fear that would come with living abroad, completely abandoning my comfort zone for a world full of unknowns, unsure if I was going to sink or swim.

It was like nothing I had ever experienced before; feelings of insecurity, doubt and incredible loneliness that became so overwhelming that, some days, I struggled to see a way through it.

I tried so hard not to let the angst beat me, to keep treading above the water, but sometimes I had to surrender and let it take control over me before I was able to take control over it. It has been these dark days, tough moments, and mental battles that have allowed me to flourish even more.

I have come to realise that home is not always a physical place or destination. It is a feeling that comes from within, a sense of true happiness and peace that only I can cultivate, and I can now say with one hundred per cent certainty that I have finally found my home.

When I look back at the little girl who tried so damn hard to be good enough for her parents, to be enough to make her mum want to live, and for her dad to want to stay, I feel so sorry for her. I want to reach out and hold her hand as I guide her along the wild journey that life is. I want to tell her that she is enough, that she doesn't need to prove herself to anyone, because the people who want to be in her life, will love and accept her for exactly who she is.

ACKNOWLEDGEMENTS

I want to start by expressing my deepest gratitude to my incredible mentor, book coach and publisher, Vanessa Barrington, the woman who believed in me from the very beginning and helped turn my dream into a reality. There is no way I could have achieved this mammoth task without you. Thank you so much.

To my amazing cover designer, Heidi Glasson and my wonderful photographer, Marili Vosmi, thank you so much for your time and incredible efforts.

To the lady who has supported me along this journey from day one, Aunty Jan, and her late husband Rex, who took on the very unexpected and incredibly huge responsibility of raising and nurturing me through the most challenging times of my life. I would not be the woman I am today without you both, and for that, I am eternally grateful.

A special thank you to Maddie for your never-ending love and support. You've stuck by me through thick and thin, and I feel so lucky to have you by my side.

I would like to thank Sam for the time we spent together. You helped me grow and flourish into a happier, stronger, and more resilient person, and you will forever hold a special place in my heart.

To my beautiful friends and personal cheer squad who have consistently supported and believed in me for as long as I have known them, Lillie, Taye, Georgia Carter, Lach, Kaisha, Alissa, Tim, Jenny and Stefan, I am truly grateful for every single one of you.

I would also like to express my greatest appreciation to my psychologist, Shannon. Thank you for always creating a safe space for me to express my deepest thoughts and emotions and for helping me work through and overcome so much.

Lastly, a special thank you to my beautiful mum. I chose to release my memoir on September 29th, the date of your anniversary, in memory of you. You may no longer be with me physically, but you will always be with me in my heart. I will never forget you. I love you.

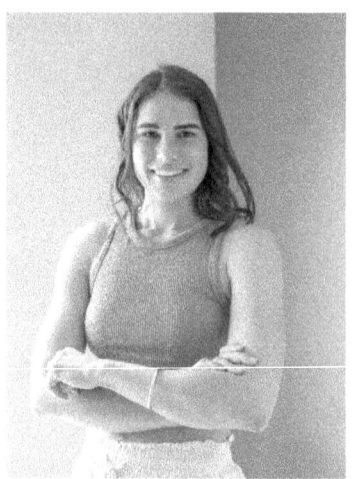

Ebonie Stirling-Gatt is an accredited Clinical Exercise Physiologist with extensive experience working with individuals with spinal cord injuries and other neurological conditions.

Ebonie is originally from sunny Gold Coast, Australia, and wrote 'Coming Home' while living and working in London and travelling the world.

When Ebonie is not writing or helping others achieve their rehabilitation goals, she can be found hiking mountain summits, exploring different cities, baking her favourite healthy recipes and spending quality time with friends.

If you have read and resonated with any part of Ebonie's story and would like some additional support through your self-healing journey, please stay in touch.

'Coming Home' is Ebonie's first novel.

Instagram: @ebonie.sg
Website: www.eboniesg.com